# PANCREATITIS DIET COOKBOOK FOR BEGINNERS

## Nourishing Meals To Ease Inflammation And Support Pancreas Health

**MOLLY MAYNARD**

# Table of contents

# Introduction

This is the "Pancreatitis Diet Cookbook for Beginners". If you or a loved one has received a pancreatitis diagnosis, you are aware of the challenges in managing this condition. Pancreatitis, a disorder marked by inflammation of the pancreas, can be excruciating and crippling, necessitating close monitoring of lifestyle and diet.

The purpose of this cookbook is to help you on your path to improved health by offering you tasty recipes and helpful advice. This book can assist you if you've recently received a diagnosis or are looking for fresh approaches to treating your symptoms.

We'll explore the definition of pancreatitis, its signs and symptoms, and how nutrition affects the condition's management in this introduction. We'll also talk about how to begin meal planning and the objectives of a pancreatitis diet.

There are many different recipes in the book that are designed to accommodate the nutritional requirements of those who have pancreatitis. There's something on these pages for everyone, from filling main courses and decadent desserts to healthy morning options.

However, this book is more than just a compilation of recipes. It's an extensive tool that will provide you the ability to take charge of your health and wellbeing. You'll discover foods that are safe for pancreatitis, cooking methods, and social gathering and dining ideas.

You can lower inflammation, ease symptoms, and enhance your general quality of life by adopting the pancreatitis diet's principles into your everyday routine. Pancreatitis might be easier to manage with the correct resources and knowledge, freeing you up to concentrate on living life to the fullest.

Now let's set off on this journey together. Flip through the pages, look through the recipes, and discover all the delectable options in the "Pancreatitis Diet Cookbook for Beginners."

# Chapter One

## Understanding Pancreatitis

Pancreatitis is inflammation in your pancreas. Although it is typically temporary (acute), it can also be a lifetime (chronic) condition. The most common symptom is abdominal pain. The most common causes are alcohol intake and gallstones

## What is pancreatitis?

Pancreatitis is inflammation in your pancreas. Inflammation causes swelling and pain. Pancreatitis can cause pain that radiates from your stomach to your back.

Your pancreas is an organ in your abdomen. It's situated between your stomach and your back.
Place your right hand over your stomach, and that's about the size and form of your pancreas.

The pancreas is in charge of regulating blood sugar levels and facilitating digestion. It creates digestive enzymes such as amylase and hormones such as insulin. The pancreatic duct transports digestive enzymes to your small intestine.

Inflammation is your immune system's response to injury. It's supposed to help heal injured tissues. The most common causes of pancreatic injuries are alcohol and gallstones obstructing the pancreatic duct.

## What are the different types of pancreatitis?

Acute and chronic pancreatitis are the two types that exist.

### Acute pancreatitis

Acute pancreatitis is a temporary condition. It occurs as your pancreas tries to heal after a minor, transient injury. Given supportive care, which includes rest, fluids, and painkillers, the majority of patients with acute pancreatitis will recover fully in a few days. On the other hand, acute pancreatitis that is really severe can result in major health issues, some of which are potentially fatal.

## Chronic pancreatitis

Chronic pancreatitis is a long-term, progressive condition. It persists and becomes worse with time. It occurs when your pancreas sustains continuous injury or damage. Eventually, though it can take years, chronic pancreatitis will cause lasting damage to your pancreatic. Your pancreas' tissues become scarred (fibrosis) as a result of ongoing inflammation, which prevents the organs from producing hormones and enzymes.

# Symptoms and Causes

## What are the symptoms of pancreatitis?

Abdominal pain is pancreatitis' main symptom.

## Additional symptoms of acute pancreatitis may include:

Nausea and vomiting.
Fast heart rate.

Fast, shallow breathing.
Fever.

**Additional symptoms of chronic pancreatitis may include:**

Indigestion and pain after eating.
Loss of appetite and unintended weight loss.
fatty feces that produce an oily residue in the restroom.
Lightheadedness (from low blood pressure).

These are signs that the breakdown of pancreatic function is starting.


## What does the pain of pancreatitis feel like?

Pancreatitis may cause abdominal pain spanning from mild to severe that may radiate to your back. Acute pancreatitis typically has a piercing character and is more severe. You might feel some tenderness in your abdomen. The degree of pain associated with chronic pancreatitis might vary. It could come and go, but it usually doesn't disappear completely. It could be more noticeable after eating. Some people have constant pain.

It may feel worse when you:

Lie flat.
Cough.
Exercise.
Eat more.

It may feel better when you:

Sit upright.
Lean forward.
Curl in a ball.
Eat less.

## Which of your symptoms point to a malfunctioning pancreas?

You will first notice changes in your digestive tract when long-term, chronic pancreatitis starts to impair pancreatic function. The breakdown and absorption of all the nutrients in your meal will be impeded if your pancreas is unable to produce and distribute its digestive enzymes. After eating, you could feel uncomfortable and start to pass undigested fats in your feces. Over time, weight loss might become evident.

## What are the most common causes of pancreatitis?

There are two primary causes of pancreatitis:

Gallstones.
Heavy drinking.

Gallstones are the most common cause of pancreatitis. An abnormal accumulation of bile, which is kept in storage in the gallbladder, results in gallstones.

The pancreas may occasionally be blocked from releasing digestive enzymes due to these gallstones. The pancreas itself begins to be eaten and damaged by these blocked enzymes, a process known as autodigestion.

Excessive alcohol intake ranks as the second most common cause. The pancreas partially metabolizes alcohol and creates harmful metabolites when consumed in high amounts.

Researchers are still trying to figure out exactly why some alcoholism sufferers get pancreatitis while most do not..

**Other causes**

Less common causes of pancreatitis include:

Infections, such as viruses.
Autoimmune disease (autoimmune pancreatitis).
Inherited gene mutations (hereditary pancreatitis).
Complications of cystic fibrosis.
High blood triglyceride levels (hypertriglyceridemia).
High blood calcium levels (hypercalcemia).
Ischemia (reduced blood supply).
Cancer.
Traumatic injury to your pancreas.
Certain medications that irritate the pancreas.

**Are the causes of chronic and acute pancreatitis the same?**

Pancreatitis is usually an acute, temporary condition. On the other hand, chronic pancreatitis can result from persistent causes, like hereditary illnesses. Chronic pancreatitis can also result from recurrent episodes of acute pancreatitis. Repetitive stress and injury can cause your pancreas to get inflamed too often, which can teach your body to stay inflamed long after the injury has healed.

**Can you die from pancreatitis?**

If your acute pancreatitis is extremely severe, you may die from its complications. A systemic reaction affecting the entire body is a rare side effect of severe acute pancreatitis. In the event that treatment is delayed, this may result in multiple organ failure and shock. If you experience symptoms of pancreatitis, you should visit the emergency hospital since you might not be able to determine how severe the condition is.

## What are the possible complications of pancreatitis?

One in five cases of acute pancreatitis is more severe, but the majority do not have any aftereffects. The reason why certain cases of severe acute pancreatitis develop and others do not is unknown. A severe case may lead to serious consequences—including death. Although they happen more gradually and don't immediately pose a threat to life, problems from chronic pancreatitis can also arise. Most complications are manageable with treatment.

**Acute pancreatitis**

Complications of severe acute pancreatitis include:

**Necrosis and infection:** In one out of three cases, severe acute pancreatitis results in the pancreatic enlarging to the point where part of the blood supply is cut off. Some parts of your pancreas experience tissue death (necrosis) due to a lack of blood supply. Bacteria roaming freely find food in necrotic (dead) tissue. Once these tissues are infected, bacteria multiply and thrive until they reach your bloodstream. Blood infection (septicemia) is an emergency. Your body initiates an immune reaction (also known as systemic inflammatory response syndrome, or SIRS) in response to an infection that enters the bloodstream. Your blood vessels may widen as a result of this immune reaction, which might lower blood pressure (septic shock) and reduce blood flow to your important organs. This can cause multiple organ failure.

**Pancreatic pseudocysts:** The pancreatic duct, which delivers pancreatic juices to your intestine, might become inflamed. This may result in tissue inflammation around the pancreas and the leakage of pancreatic fluids. A pseudocyst is a rigid capsule that surrounds the fluid and develops over time from the inflammatory area. Many pseudocysts don't require medical attention or create symptoms. However, on rare occasions, they may become infected or grow to a size that is uncomfortable. In rare cases, a blood vessel may erode into a pseudocyst, causing internal bleeding in the cyst. In these situations, your medical professional might have to step in to stop the bleeding or empty the cyst.

**Chronic pancreatitis:** Chronic pancreatitis can result from recurrent episodes of acute pancreatitis. Your pancreas's constant inflammation eventually causes the tissues to scar (fibrosis). Your pancreas's fibrosis prevents it from functioning as a gland. It creates progressively fewer of the hormones and enzymes your body requires over time, which causes more issues.


**Chronic pancreatitis**

Over time, complications from chronic pancreatitis might arise and include:

**Exocrine pancreatic insufficiency (EPI), malabsorption and malnutrition:** Your pancreas generates fewer and fewer of the enzymes your digestive system needs as the fibrosis in it deepens.  This results in the small intestine becoming less able to absorb nutrients, particularly fats and fat-soluble vitamins.  Excess fats make their way through your feces, leading to fatty stools and eventually chronic diarrhea. You could start to lose weight and eventually experience the impacts of the missing nutrients as your body absorbs less nutrition from your food.

**Hypoglycemia, hyperglycemia and Type 1 diabetes:** Your pancreas will also generate fewer hormones that control your blood sugar (glucose) if you have chronic pancreatitis. You may have symptoms from either a lack of insulin, which produces hyperglycemia (high blood sugar), or a lack of glucagon, which causes hypoglycemia (low blood sugar), depending on which is impacted first. Diabetes eventually arises when both hormone supplies are exhausted.

**Chronic pain:** While some individuals with chronic pancreatitis never suffer pain or eventually experience a remission of discomfort, others eventually get severe pain that never goes away. Even with medicine, it can be difficult to manage and have an impact on your mental health.

**Increased risk of pancreatic cancer:** Chronic inflammation is a risk factor for cancer wherever it occurs. In people with chronic pancreatitis, the risk of pancreatic adenocarcinoma is between 1% and 2%. The symptoms may be missed because they resemble those of chronic pancreatitis. It is advised by physicians that patients with persistent pancreatitis have routine cancer screenings.

# Diagnosis and Tests

## How is pancreatitis diagnosed?

Your doctor will examine your pancreas using imaging and blood testing if you exhibit typical pancreatitis symptoms. A pancreas blood test checks your blood for higher than normal amounts of pancreatic enzymes. If the levels are three times higher than normal, pancreatitis will be suspected by your healthcare professional. A MRI or CT scan, or another cross-sectional imaging test, may be used to confirm the diagnosis. These tests may reveal other anomalies in addition to pancreatic enlargement and fluid accumulation.

Your healthcare practitioner might prescribe more testing if they think you have chronic pancreatitis, such as:

**Glucose test:** to ascertain whether your pancreas is still producing adequate insulin.

**Stool elastase test:** to determine whether your pancreas is producing adequate digestive enzymes.

**Fecal fat analysis:** to check for signs of fat malabsorption, such as extra fat in the feces.

**Blood tests:** to determine whether your blood has adequate fat-soluble vitamins and to evaluate your nutritional condition.

# Management and Treatment

### How is pancreatitis treated?

The cause, severity, and duration of the condition all influence the course of treatment. In general, if you have pancreatitis symptoms, you should consult a doctor at once. Depending on what triggered the illness and how bad it is, some cases of acute pancreatitis may resolve on their own. Most patients with acute pancreatitis will require pain medication to get through it in the interim. For certain causes, some people will require emergency care. Moreover, some will require intensive care due to complications

### Acute pancreatitis

Treatment for acute pancreatitis may include:

**Supportive care**

In cases when the underlying cause of your pancreatitis has been identified and treated, the focus of your care will be on promoting your body's natural healing mechanism. This usually includes:

**IV fluids:** Hydration is crucial for healing since pancreatitis dehydrates the body.

**Tube feeding:** To assist you get enough nutrition if you can't take meals by mouth, your doctors might give you food through a tube inserted into your stomach or nose.

**Parenteral nutrition:** Your doctors might decide to use an intravenous line to deliver nutrients in extremely severe situations.

**Pain relief:** You will receive medication orally or via an IV that enters your bloodstream directly.

**Gallstone removal**

Your doctor might have to remove an affected gallstone from your bile ducts if you have gallstone pancreatitis. Additionally, they will advise gallbladder removal surgery to keep gallstones from bothering you in the future. Procedures may include:

**Endoscopic retrograde:**
cholangiopancreatography (ERCP): During this treatment, an endoscope—a tiny, flexible catheter with a camera attached—is used to see inside your bile ducts. This method works for the majority of gallstones that are in your bile ducts. The endoscope enters your stomach and bile ducts after passing down your mouth and into your esophagus. Images are sent to a monitor by it. The endoscopist can remove gallstones by inserting tools through the catheter while keeping an eye on the monitor.

**Gallbladder removal surgery:** The likelihood of gallstones bothering you again is rather significant if they have already sent you to the hospital. The usual course of treatment for gallstones that create problems is gallbladder removal. Usually, minimally invasive (laparoscopic) surgery can be used to do it. Using a laparoscope, a few tiny incisions are made to remove your gallbladder during a laparoscopic cholecystectomy. One of the incisions is used to install a tiny camera. Depending on their condition, some patients can need open surgery.

**Additional support**

If things get complicated, you could also require:

- Antibiotics.
- Procedures to eliminate dead tissue or drain fluid.
- Intensive care.

**Chronic pancreatitis**

You can be referred to a gastroenterologist by your general practitioner if you have chronic pancreatitis. In order to slow down the disease's course and control discomfort, the first line of treatment for chronic pancreatitis involves making lifestyle modifications. In the end, insulin injections and enzyme supplements could be necessary to replenish the insulin and enzymes your pancreas is no longer able to produce.

## Lifestyle changes

It's imperative that you give up smoking and alcohol if you have chronic pancreatitis. These variables both have a significant role in the progression of pancreatitis and will hasten the illness's course. Your medical professional can connect you with resources to support your quitting. Maintaining a low-fat diet rich in fruits and vegetables and consuming lots of water each day are also crucial.

## Pain management

Long-term pain management can be complex. To determine which treatments and medications are most effective for you, you might need to try a range of options. It's important to communicate with your healthcare practitioner about your discomfort, particularly if you're not getting better on your own. To assist you in managing your pain, they may refer you to a chronic pain specialist. Your symptoms may occasionally be relieved by endoscopic treatments to remove pancreatic stones or scar tissue. For certain people, another alternative is to inject local anesthetics into the pancreatic nerves (a procedure known as a celiac plexus block).

**Supplements**

Exocrine pancreatic insufficiency (EPI) is a condition that many people with chronic pancreatitis may eventually acquire. These individuals will require pancreatic enzyme supplements. In order to consume enough calories and micronutrients (vitamins and minerals), you might also need to take nutritional supplements. Some people will eventually become insulin dependent as a result of glucose intolerance and diabetes.

**Surgery**

Your doctor may recommend surgery to remove a portion of your pancreas (resection) if there is severe inflammation concentrated in one area and it is causing unbearable discomfort or complications. They may advise removing your pancreas entirely (total pancreatectomy) in extremely severe situations where it is still causing you a great deal of pain despite the damage.

# Prevention

**How can I prevent pancreatitis?**

While you cannot prevent every cause, you can lower your risk by consuming alcohol in moderation. By lowering cholesterol, you can lower your chance of gallstones, which is the other major cause. If you've experienced acute pancreatitis, giving up alcohol and cigarettes can help keep it from happening again. Removing your gallbladder can stop a recurrence of gallstone pancreatitis.

# Chapter Two

## Importance of diet in managing pancreatitis

The human body functions similarly to a sophisticated, well-tuned machine, with each organ contributing uniquely to the preservation of general health. In this intricate symphony of our body's functions, the pancreas plays a pivotal role. This little, leaf-shaped organ, which is located behind your stomach, helps with digestion and is in charge of controlling blood sugar levels.

However, the body's delicate equilibrium can be upset when the pancreas becomes inflamed, a condition known as pancreatitis. In the quest for effective Pancreatitis treatment, one factor acts as a beacon of hope: Nutrition. In this book, you will learn how a balanced diet plays a major role in the treatment of pancreatitis. Keep reading to find out how food can become medicine.

# The role of nutrition in pancreatitis treatment

Imagine that your body is a battleground and your immune system is the army. In this scenario, nutrition serves as the weapon that fortifies your immune system to combat inflammation and promote healing. A balanced diet can have a big impact on how quickly you recover from pancreatitis and how well you feel overall.

**Reduces digestive stress**

Simple-to-digest foods like whole grains, lean meats, and steamed veggies are part of a diet that is rich in nutrients. By following a pancreatitis-friendly diet, you get essential vitamins and proteins without burdening your pancreas, allowing the organ to heal without unnecessary strain.

**Keeps your body hydrated**

Staying well-hydrated is essential for individuals battling pancreatitis. It supports digestion, helps the body eliminate toxins, and maintains overall health.

**Micronutrients act as your
anti-inflammatory allies**

Foods high in nutrients have powerful
anti-inflammatory components that can aid in
the battle against pancreatic inflammation.
Zinc helps with tissue regeneration, vitamin D
strengthens the immune system, vitamin C,
with its antioxidant qualities, can lower
inflammation, and omega-3 fatty acids help
with healing.

**Balancing blood sugar**

Blood sugar levels can be severely affected by
pancreatitis, which is especially dangerous for
those who already have diabetes. Adopting a
diet that is rich in low-glycemic foods, such
berries, nuts, and leafy greens can help
patients control their blood sugar levels and
assist the pancreas in regulating insulin.

## How can foods affect your pancreas?

If you have pancreatitis, you might be
wondering what meals are beneficial. The
digestive enzymes protease, amylin, and
lipase, which break down proteins,

carbohydrates, and fats, respectively, are secreted by the pancreas to aid in the breakdown of the food you ingest.

To properly break down food, the pancreas releases a lot of enzymes when a heavy meal, such a fatty pizza, is consumed.
Furthermore, the pancreas must release insulin in order to control the blood sugar reaction to the meal because the pizza is high in carbohydrates.

**Foods for a pancreatitis diet**

Try to incorporate the following types of food:

Lean-meat proteins
White fish or canned fish
Beans and lentils
Whole grains
Fruits and vegetables
Low-fat dairy
Fresh herbs and spices

Even though they're healthy, avocado, olive oil, fatty fish, nuts and seeds should only be consumed in moderation as they are heavy in fat.

# Nutrition treatment for pancreatitis

Nutrition is crucial in the management of pancreatitis because the pancreas is heavily involved in digestion.
Giving the pancreas time to rest is the main strategy for treating acute pancreatitis. This could entail a brief period of fasting during which you only consume liquids.

You may go towards a diet that is low in fat and concentrated sugars as your symptoms get better in order to lessen the strain on your pancreas. This may be all that is needed to treat acute pancreatitis because the illness only lasts a short time.
Sometimes, carefully tailored nutrition can be provided through tube feeding to individuals who are at risk of malnutrition without causing injury to the pancreas.

Parenteral nutrition, also referred to as intravenous nutrition, is necessary in rare instances where no food is tolerated for a prolonged period of time.

Those who have chronic pancreatitis make significant dietary changes as part of their lifestyle. Consuming a healthy diet can assist to slow down the damage caused by chronic pancreatitis and maintain the pancreas functioning as best as it can, even though the damage cannot be undone.

When it comes to managing nutrition in chronic pancreatitis, there are numerous priorities:

**Preventing malnutrition**

There is a considerable risk of nutrient deficiencies due to decreased food absorption, decreased appetite, discomfort after eating, and elevated inflammatory energy requirements.

**Reducing strain on the pancreas**

Heavy meals, particularly those high in fats and carbohydrates, will cause the pancreas to work harder and create more digestive enzymes. It's critical to limit certain nutrients—but not avoiding them entirely—in order to lower pancreatic inflammation. If pancreatic enzymes are required, they must be taken with every

meal and snack in order to support the
pancreas during digestion.

**Controlling blood sugar**

Keep in mind that a damaged pancreas might
not be able to meet the body's needs for blood
sugar. Modest diet adjustments, particularly in
the areas of portion control and moderation of
carbohydrates, can aid in the regulation of
blood sugar levels.

**Avoiding alcohol**

Drinking too much alcohol can aggravate
pancreatitis and induce discomfort right away.
When pancreatitis is present, alcohol should be
completely avoided.

What does a pancreatitis diet actually entail,
keeping these principles in mind?

# What is the best diet for pancreatitis?

A pancreatitis diet includes the following
components:

## Small, frequent meals

Since smaller meal portions are easier for the pancreas to process, they are typically better accepted. Eating frequently also helps to prevent malnutrition. Try to have six meals a day.

## Moderate to low fat

You will want to keep total fat to about 30% of total calories. All forms of fat are included in this, even healthy fats like olive oil. For the purpose of gauging how much total fat you typically consume, it could be a good idea to record all of your meals for a few days.

## Consider MCT oil

Medium-chain triglycerides, or MCTs, are a form of fat that may be absorbed without the help of pancreatic enzymes. Based on certain research, these oils may be more tolerable and may help with pancreatitis-related diarrhea. MCT is available as a supplement.

### High-quality lean protein

Protein is important for healing and maintaining strength. In a low-fat diet for pancreatitis, it is crucial to give priority to lean protein options like turkey, fish, chicken, or plant sources because many protein sources also include fat.

### Plenty of fruits and vegetables

Try to fill half of your plate with vegetables and fruits. By doing this, vitamin and mineral requirements will be satisfied. In addition, they have phytochemicals, antioxidants, and other anti-inflammatory substances. Additionally, fiber from fruits and vegetables helps prevent blood sugar rises.

### Less Processed foods

In general, processed foods have poor nutrient quality, high sugar, fat, and sodium content, and low fiber content. Making whole, unprocessed food choices is a crucial component of the pancreatitis diet.

## Select the right Carbohydrate Types and Amounts

Carbohydrates (sugars and starches) are an essential energy source, and they generally should make up about 50% of the total calories. However, not all carbohydrates are created equal. Because they contain more fiber and nutrients, whole grains are recommended.

## Avoid too much-added sugar

Sugars that are added to food are those that are not found naturally in it; they can easily lead to overindulgence in sugar without the consumer realizing it. Sodas, sports drinks, juices, candies, pastries, and a variety of other items all include added sugars. To obtain the most accurate information, consult the nutrition facts label.

## Adequate fluids

A sometimes disregarded but equally crucial component of diet is staying hydrated. It is advised to consume 8 to 10 glasses of fluid per day. If you suffer from dehydration, think about carrying a reusable water bottle as a reminder.

# Pancreatitis diet food list

Below are list of foods to eat when you have pancreatitis:

**Fruits and vegetables:**

- Apple
- Blueberries
- Raspberries
- Orange
- Banana
- Spinach
- Cauliflower
- Broccoli
- Tomato
- Green Beans

A pancreatitis diet plan can include most fruits and vegetables because they are generally well-tolerated. A grapefruit is an exception, as it can interfere with a lot of medications. If grapefruit is a regular in your diet, consult your physician.

**Starches:**

- Potato
- Sweet Potato
- Brown rice
- Whole wheat bread
- Whole wheat pasta
- Black beans
- Oatmeal
- Corn

**Meats/proteins:**

- Skinless chicken breast
- Skinless turkey breast
- Fish
- Egg whites
- Whole egg (1-2 per day)
- Tofu
- Protein powder

**Fats (limit overall fat):**

- Olive oil
- Oil sprays
- MCT oil
- Almonds
- Cashews
- Peanuts

- Walnuts
- Seeds
- low-fat cottage cheese

**Beverages:**

- Water
- Skim or 1% milk
- Sugar-free seltzer water

## Foods to avoid with pancreatitis

Eat as little of the following foods as you can. Remember that this is not an exhaustive list, and base your dietary decisions on the aforementioned principles.

- Sausages
- Processed meats like roast beef, pepperoni, and salami.
- High-fat red meats, like burgers and ribeye steak.
- Fried foods, including french fries.
- Processed cheeses with a lot of fat, like American and cheddar.
- Bacon
- Butter

- Cream soups
- Whole milk
- Ice-cream
- Candy
- Soda
- Juice
- Sports drinks
- Alcohol
- Sugary cereal
- Chocolate
- Avocado

# Chapter Three

## Getting started with the pancreatitis diet

If you've been diagnosed with chronic pancreatitis, adopting a low-fat diet and stopping alcohol is essential for managing your condition and reducing symptoms. To manage your pain, you can also take medication. Making changes like these may seem hard. Planning, consulting your physician, and enlisting the help of loved ones can help make these adjustments possible.

## Getting started with meal planning:

Consult with a healthcare professional or registered dietitian who specializes in pancreatitis to create a personalized meal plan that meets your individual dietary needs and preferences.

Start by gradually eliminating trigger foods from your diet, such as fried foods, fatty meats, processed snacks, and alcohol.

Focus on incorporating pancreatitis-friendly foods into your meals, including lean proteins, whole grains, fruits, vegetables, and low-fat dairy products.

Experiment with different cooking techniques, such as baking, grilling, steaming, and sautéing, to prepare delicious and nutritious meals without adding excess fat.

Keep a food journal to track your symptoms and identify any potential trigger foods or patterns that may worsen your pancreatitis symptoms.

## How can you care for yourself at home?

Do not drink alcohol. In addition to potentially aggravating your discomfort, it might also lead to additional issues, such as worsening pancreatic swelling. In case you require assistance in quitting, let your physician know.

Support groups, counseling, and medication
can help you stay sober at times.

See your doctor if taking pancreatic enzyme
supplements is necessary to aid in the
breakdown of protein and fat by your body.

**Eat a low-fat diet**

Attempt to replace your three major meals a
day with four to six smaller meals and snacks.

**Choose lean meats.**

- Cut off all fat you can see.

- Consume poultry such as chicken, duck,
  and turkey, skinless

- Omega-3 fat is found in a variety of fish,
  including salmon, lake trout, tuna, and
  herring. However, stay away from
  oil-canned fish, such as sardines in olive
  oil.

- Instead of frying meats, poultry, or fish in
  butter or lard, bake, broil, or grill them.

Every day, consume non-fat or low-fat milk, cheese, yogurt, or other milk products.

- Check cheese labels and select low-fat varieties.

- Try yogurt, cream cheese, or sour cream that are fat free

- Try fortified soy beverage.

- Steer clear of cream soups and pasta sauces.

- Eat low-fat ice cream, frozen yogurt, or sorbet. Avoid regular ice cream.

Eat a variety of vegetables and fruits. They are nutrient-dense and low in fat.

Consume whole grain pasta, rice, crackers, breads, and cereals. Steer clear of breads that have been deep-fried or fried, such as croissants and bannocks, as well as breads with a lot of fat.

Find out how to bake and cook with less sugar and fat.

Use herbs and spices (such mint, tarragon, or basil), fat-free sauces, or lemon juice to season your food.

To replace part or all of the fat when baking, try applesauce, prune puree, or mashed bananas.

Use no more than one tablespoon of fats and oils per meal, such as butter, margarine, mayonnaise, and salad dressing.

**Avoid high-fat foods, such as:**

- Egg yolks, chocolate, ice cream, whole milk, and processed cheese.
- Fried, deep fried, or buttered foods.
- Sausage, salami, and bacon.
- Cakes, pies, cookies, cinnamon buns, and other pastries.
- Prepared munchies such as potato chips, granola and nut bars, and mixed nuts.
- Avocado with coconut.
- Meals from fast food and convenience stores are often high in fat.

To determine serving sizes and ingredients, learn to read food labels.

# Diet tips

In order to minimize discomfort and stop the illness from coming back, your doctor will typically advise you to adhere to a specific diet while you heal from acute pancreatitis.

The dietary requirements of individuals with acute and chronic pancreatitis may differ.

Malnutrition may be more likely to occur in those with chronic pancreatitis. This is due to the possibility that chronic pancreatitis may impair the body's ability to absorb nutrients from food. Helping you receive sufficient nutrients from your diet may be the main focus of advice if you have chronic pancreatitis.

Vitamins A, D, E, and K Trusted Source are most commonly found to be lacking as a result of chronic pancreatitis.

In the event that you have pancreatitis, always see your physician or nutritionist before making any dietary changes. These are some recommendations they might make:

Consume five to six modest meals daily to aid in pancreatitis recovery. Compared to eating multiple large meals, this can be less of a burden on your digestive system.

You might want to refrain from consuming too much fiber at once if you have acute pancreatitis. Before reintroducing high-fiber whole grains, you might want to start with soft, starchy carbohydrates like bread, potatoes, and pasta to give your digestive system time to heal.

A high-fiber diet may need to be avoided by some individuals who have chronic pancreatitis. When you have this disease, eating a lot of fiber may reduce the efficiency of your digestive enzymes.

Consult your physician or a dietitian about keeping an eye on your vitamin levels if you have been diagnosed with chronic pancreatitis. If a person can't get enough nutrients from their food, they might need to take supplements.

## Signs your pancreas is struggling

These are a few typical indicators of pancreatic diseases that you should not overlook:

- Irregular blood sugar levels
- Digestive problems, like bloating or excessive gas
- Unhealthy weight
- Jaundice, or the yellowing of the eyes or skin,
- Unusual color of the stool; normally, brown stools show a healthy pancreas.
- Abdominal pain or ongoing stomach ache

**Setting realistic goals:**

When managing pancreatitis through diet, setting realistic goals is crucial for long-term success and adherence.

**Understand your condition:** Before setting goals, it's essential to have a clear understanding of your pancreatitis and how it affects your body. Educate yourself about the causes, symptoms, and dietary recommendations for pancreatitis. Consult with your healthcare provider or a registered dietitian to gain insights into your specific condition and dietary needs.

**Focus on small, incremental changes:** Instead of trying to overhaul your diet overnight, focus on making small, sustainable changes over time. Start by identifying one or two dietary habits that you'd like to improve, such as reducing your intake of high-fat foods or increasing your consumption of fruits and vegetables. Once you've successfully incorporated these changes into your routine, gradually add more goals as you progress.

**Be specific and measurable:** When setting goals, be specific about what you want to achieve and how you'll measure your progress. For example, instead of setting a vague goal like "eat healthier," set a specific goal such as "eat at least two servings of vegetables with lunch and dinner each day." This facilitates keeping track of your development and maintaining motivation.

**Set realistic timeframes:** While it's important to challenge yourself, it's also crucial to set goals that are achievable within a realistic timeframe. Consider your current lifestyle, commitments, and dietary preferences when setting deadlines for your goals. Instead of anticipating quick fixes, strive for steady progress.

**Celebrate your successes:** Celebrate your achievements, no matter how small they may seem. Recognize and reward yourself for reaching milestones along the way, whether it's trying a new pancreatitis-friendly recipe, sticking to your meal plan for a week straight, or successfully navigating a social event while adhering to your dietary restrictions.

**Adjust as needed:** Be flexible and willing to adjust your goals as needed based on your progress and changing circumstances. Don't give up if you run into challenges or setbacks. Use them as learning opportunities and reassess your goals to ensure they remain realistic and attainable.

**Creating a meal plan:**

A well-designed meal plan is an essential tool for managing pancreatitis and ensuring that you're following a pancreatitis-friendly diet.

**Assess your dietary needs:** Start by assessing your current dietary habits and identifying areas for improvement. Consider any food intolerances, allergies, or sensitivities you may have, as well as any specific recommendations from your healthcare provider or dietitian regarding your pancreatitis.

**Set meal times:** Establish regular meal times and aim to eat every 3-4 hours throughout the day to help stabilize blood sugar levels and prevent overeating. Consistency in meal timing can also help regulate digestive function and reduce the risk of pancreatitis flare-ups.

**Balance your plate:** When planning your meals, aim for a balanced combination of macronutrients (carbohydrates, proteins, and fats) to support overall health and digestion. Arrange your plate so that non-starchy veggies make up half of it, lean protein sources make up a quarter, and whole grains or starchy vegetables make up the other quarter.

**Incorporate pancreatitis-friendly foods:** Choose foods that are low in fat, easy to digest, and gentle on the pancreas. Focus on incorporating lean proteins such as poultry, fish, tofu, and legumes, as well as whole grains, fruits, and vegetables. Avoid or limit high-fat foods, fried foods, processed meats, and alcohol.

**Plan for snacks:** Include healthy snacks between meals to keep your energy levels stable and prevent excessive hunger. Opt for nutrient-dense snacks such as fresh fruit, raw vegetables with hummus, Greek yogurt, or a handful of nuts and seeds.

**Variety and flexibility:** Keep your meals interesting and enjoyable by incorporating a variety of flavors, textures, and cuisines. Experiment with different recipes, ingredients, and cooking techniques to keep things exciting. Be flexible with your meal plan and allow for occasional indulgences while staying mindful of your overall dietary goals.

**Preparation and batch cooking:** Set aside time each week for meal preparation and batch cooking to streamline your meal plan and save time during busy weekdays. Prepare larger batches of staple foods such as grains, proteins, and vegetables that can be portioned out and reheated throughout the week.

**Listen to your body:** Observe how your body reacts to various foods and modify your diet

plan as necessary. Keep a food journal to track
your symptoms and identify any potential
trigger foods or patterns that may worsen your
pancreatitis symptoms.

# Chapter Four

## Pancreatitis-friendly ingredients and cooking techniques

### Low-fat cooking methods

Low-fat cooking methods are essential for individuals managing pancreatitis, as they help reduce the strain on the pancreas and minimize symptoms. Here are some low-fat cooking methods to consider incorporating into your meal preparation:

**Grilling:** Grilling is a fantastic way to cook lean proteins such as chicken, fish, and turkey without adding extra fat. Marinate your protein in herbs, spices, and citrus juices for added flavor, then grill until cooked through.

**Baking:** Baking is a gentle cooking method that requires minimal added fat. Use a non-stick cooking spray or line your baking dish with parchment paper to prevent sticking. You can bake a variety of foods, including vegetables, fish, poultry, and even desserts like fruit crisps or baked apples.

**Steaming:** Steaming is one of the healthiest cooking methods, as it preserves the nutrients in foods without the need for added fats. Simply place your ingredients in a steamer basket over boiling water and cook until tender. Steamed vegetables, fish, and dumplings are all delicious options.

**Boiling:** Boiling is a simple and effective way to cook foods without adding fat. Use water or low-sodium broth as your cooking liquid and add herbs, spices, and aromatics for flavor. Boil pasta, rice, grains, and vegetables until tender, then drain and serve.

**Poaching:** Poaching involves cooking foods gently in simmering liquid, such as water, broth, or wine. It's an excellent method for cooking delicate proteins like chicken breasts, fish fillets, or eggs. Poached chicken can be shredded and used in salads, sandwiches, or wraps.

**Stir-frying**: While traditional stir-frying often uses oil, you can adapt this cooking method by using a minimal amount of oil or cooking spray and cooking over high heat for a short period. Stir-fry lean proteins, vegetables, and tofu for a quick and flavorful meal.

**Broiling:** Broiling is similar to grilling but cooks food from above rather than below. It's a great way to cook lean cuts of meat, poultry, and fish quickly and with minimal added fat. Keep an eye on your food to prevent burning, and flip halfway through cooking for even browning.

**Microwaving:** Microwaving is a convenient cooking method that requires little to no added fat. Use microwave-safe dishes to cook vegetables, grains, and proteins quickly and efficiently. Just be sure to cover your food to prevent splattering and stir occasionally for even cooking.

## Substitutions and Swaps

Making substitutions and swaps in your recipes can help you create pancreatitis-friendly meals without sacrificing flavor. Here are some ideas for substituting ingredients to make your recipes more gentle on the pancreas:

**Replace High-Fat Meats:**
Swap fatty cuts of meat like beef brisket or pork ribs for leaner options such as skinless chicken breast, turkey, or lean cuts of beef like sirloin or tenderloin.

**Use Low-Fat Dairy Alternatives:**
Go for skim or low-fat milk instead of whole milk.
Choose plain, unsweetened Greek yogurt or lactose-free yogurt over full-fat varieties.
Replace regular cottage cheese with low-fat cottage cheese.

**Choose Healthy Fats:**
Use small amounts of heart-healthy fats like olive oil or avocado oil for cooking instead of butter or lard.
Incorporate nuts and seeds like almonds, walnuts, or chia seeds into recipes for added texture and flavor.

**Swap High-Fat Cooking Methods:**
Instead of frying foods in oil, try baking, grilling, steaming, or broiling them for a lower-fat option.
Use non-stick cooking spray or parchment paper to prevent sticking when baking or roasting foods.

**Reduce Added Sugars:**
Cut back on added sugars by using natural
sweeteners like honey, maple syrup, or stevia
in moderation.
Go for unsweetened applesauce or mashed
ripe bananas as natural sweeteners in baking
recipes.

**Choose Whole Grains:**
Replace refined grains with whole grains like
brown rice, quinoa, oats, or whole wheat pasta
for added fiber and nutrients.

**Experiment with Low-FODMAP Foods:**
If you're following a low-FODMAP diet, explore
substitutions for high-FODMAP ingredients like
onions, garlic, and wheat-based products.
Use green onions (green parts only),
garlic-infused oil, or garlic-infused broth for
flavor without the FODMAPs.

**Incorporate Flavorful Herbs and Spices:**
Add depth of flavor to dishes with herbs and
spices like basil, cilantro, ginger, turmeric,
cumin, and cinnamon instead of relying on
added fats or sauces.

**Choose Low-Sodium Options:**
Go for low-sodium or no-salt-added versions of
canned foods like beans, broth, and canned
vegetables to reduce sodium intake.

**Explore Plant-Based Proteins:**
Incorporate plant-based proteins like tofu,
tempeh, lentils, and beans into your meals as
alternatives to high-fat animal proteins.

# Social gathering and dining ideas

Navigating social gatherings and dining out can
be challenging when managing pancreatitis,
but with some preparation and creativity, it's
possible to enjoy these occasions while
sticking to your dietary restrictions. Here are
some ideas for social gathering and dining:

**Communicate Your Dietary Needs:** Don't be
afraid to communicate your dietary needs to
your host or the restaurant staff in advance. Let
them know about your pancreatitis and any
specific dietary restrictions you have. Most
hosts and restaurants will be happy to
accommodate your needs.

**Bring a Dish:** If you're attending a potluck-style gathering, consider bringing a dish that you know is pancreatitis-friendly. This ensures that you'll have at least one option that you can enjoy without worrying about triggering symptoms.

**Focus on Simple, Whole Foods:** When dining out, look for simple, whole foods that are less likely to exacerbate pancreatitis symptoms. Choose grilled or baked proteins, steamed vegetables, and plain starches like rice or baked potatoes.

**Avoid Fried and Greasy Foods:** Fried and greasy foods can be hard to digest and may worsen pancreatitis symptoms. Avoid dishes that are deep-fried or cooked in heavy sauces or oils.

**Ask for Modifications:** Don't hesitate to ask for modifications to menu items to make them more pancreatitis-friendly. For example, ask for sauces or dressings on the side, request grilled instead of fried preparation, or substitute high-fat sides for healthier options like steamed vegetables or a side salad.

**Be Mindful of Portion Sizes:** Pay attention to portion sizes when dining out, as large portions can be overwhelming for the digestive system. Consider splitting an entree with a dining companion or asking for a half portion if available.

**Stay Hydrated:** Drink plenty of water throughout the gathering or meal to stay hydrated and aid digestion. Avoid sugary or alcoholic beverages, as they can irritate the pancreas and worsen symptoms.

**Choose Low-FODMAP Options:** If you're following a low-FODMAP diet, look for menu items that are naturally low in fermentable carbohydrates. Go for grilled proteins, plain rice or potatoes, and non-creamy sauces or dressings.

**Listen to Your Body:** Pay attention to how your body reacts to different foods and adjust your choices accordingly. If you start to experience symptoms like abdominal pain or discomfort, take a break from eating and give your digestive system time to rest.

**Focus on Enjoying the Company:**
Remember there are other reasons to attend social events besides the cuisine. Focus on enjoying the company of friends and loved ones, and don't let dietary restrictions overshadow the joy of being together.

# Chapter Five

## Pancreatitis-friendly breakfast recipes

### Low-FODMAP Banana Oat Pancakes

**Ingredients:**

- 1 ripe banana, mashed
- 1 cup old-fashioned rolled oats
- 2 eggs
- 1/4 teaspoon cinnamon
- 1/4 teaspoon vanilla extract (optional)
- Non-stick cooking spray or olive oil for cooking
- Fresh berries or sliced banana for serving (optional)

**Preparation:**

- In a mixing bowl, combine the mashed banana, rolled oats, eggs, cinnamon, and vanilla extract (if using).

- Mix until well combined.

- Let the batter rest for 5-10 minutes to allow the oats to absorb some moisture and thicken.

- Heat a non-stick skillet or griddle over medium heat and lightly coat with cooking spray or olive oil.

- Turn about 1/4 cup of the pancake batter onto the skillet for each pancake.

- Allow to cook for two to three minutes, or until the edges start to firm and bubbles appear on the surface.

- Turn the pancakes and cook for an additional 1-2 minutes, or until golden brown and cooked through.

- Repeat with the remaining batter, adding more cooking spray or oil to the skillet as needed.

- Serve the pancakes warm, topped with fresh berries or sliced banana if desired.

**Cooking Time:** 15 minutes

**Number of Servings:** Makes approximately 8 small pancakes

**Nutritional Information (per serving, without toppings):**

- Calories: 80
- Total Fat: 2g
    - Saturated Fat: 0.5g
    - Trans Fat: 0g
- Cholesterol: 47mg
- Sodium: 21mg
- Total Carbohydrates: 13g
    - Dietary Fiber: 2g
    - Sugars: 3g
- Protein: 3g

**Banana Oat Breakfast Muffins**

**Ingredients:**

- 2 ripe bananas, mashed
- 2 cups old-fashioned rolled oats
- 1/4 cup of almond milk (or any other non-dairy milk of your choice)
- 2 tablespoons maple syrup (optional)
- 1 teaspoon vanilla extract
- 1 teaspoon cinnamon
- 1/2 teaspoon baking powder

- Pinch of salt
- Chopped nuts, dried fruits, or dark chocolate chips (optional add-ins)

**Preparation:**

- Preheat the oven to 350°F (175°C)

- A muffin tin should be greased with oil or line with paper liners.

- In a mixing bowl, combine the mashed bananas, almond milk, maple syrup (if using), and vanilla extract.

- Add the rolled oats, cinnamon, baking powder, and salt to the bowl and mix until well combined.

- Add any optional add-ins, such chopped almonds or dark chocolate chips, and mix them in.

- Using a spoon, scoop the batter into each muffin tin, filling it to about 3/4 full.

- The muffins should be baked for 20 to 25 minutes, or until they are golden brown and a toothpick inserted in the center comes out clean.

- For a few minutes, let the muffins cool in the tin before moving them to a wire rack to completely cool off.

**Cooking Time:** 20-25 minutes

**Number of Servings:** 12 muffins

**Nutritional Information (per muffin):**

- Calories: 110
- Total Fat: 2g
    - Saturated Fat: 0.3g
- Cholesterol: 0mg
- Sodium: 39mg
- Total Carbohydrates: 22g
    - Dietary Fiber: 3g
    - Sugars: 6g
- Protein: 3g

**Vegetable Omelette**

**Ingredients:**

- 2 eggs
- 1/4 cup diced bell peppers

- 1/4 cup diced tomatoes
- 1/4 cup chopped spinach
- Salt and pepper to taste
- 1 teaspoon olive oil

**Preparation:**

- Mix the eggs until well combined in a small bowl.

- Season with salt and pepper.

- The olive oil should be heated in a non-stick skillet over medium heat.

- Combine the diced bell peppers and sauté for 2-3 minutes until slightly softened.

- Add the diced tomatoes and chopped spinach to the skillet and cook for another 1-2 minutes until the vegetables are heated through.

- Pour the beaten eggs over the vegetables in the skillet, tilting the pan to spread them evenly.

- Cook the omelette for 2-3 minutes until the edges begin to set.

- Carefully flip the omelette and cook for another 1-2 minutes until cooked through.

- Transfer the omelette onto a plate and serve hot.

**Cooking Time:** 5-7 minutes

**Number of Servings:** 1

**Nutritional Information (per serving):**

- Calories: 220
- Total Fat: 15g
    - Saturated Fat: 4g
- Cholesterol: 370mg
- Sodium: 280mg
- Total Carbohydrates: 9g
    - Dietary Fiber: 3g
    - Sugars: 5g
- Protein: 14g

**Greek Yogurt with Berries and Almonds**

**Ingredients:**

- 1/2 cup low-fat or non-fat plain greek yogurt
- 1/4 cup mixed berries (like blueberries, strawberries, raspberries)
- 1 tablespoon sliced almonds
- 1 teaspoon honey (optional)

**Preparation:**

- Using a spoon, scoop the Greek yogurt into a bowl or serving dish.

- Top with mixed berries and sliced almonds.

- If desired, drizzle with honey.

- Serve immediately.

**Preparation Time:** 2 minutes

**Number of Servings:** 1

**Nutritional Information (per serving):**

- Calories: 180
- Total Fat: 7g
  - Saturated Fat: 0.5g
- Cholesterol: 10mg
- Sodium: 50mg
- Total Carbohydrates: 17g
  - Dietary Fiber: 3g
  - Sugars: 11g
- Protein: 15g

**Quinoa Breakfast Bowl**

**Ingredients:**

- 1/2 cup cooked quinoa
- 1/4 cup sliced strawberries
- 1/4 cup sliced banana
- 1 tablespoon chopped nuts (like almonds, walnuts)
- 1 tablespoon honey (optional)
- Pinch of cinnamon

**Preparation:**

- In a bowl, combine the cooked quinoa, sliced strawberries, sliced banana, and chopped nuts.

- Drizzle with honey and sprinkle with cinnamon.

- Mix gently to combine.

- Serve immediately.

**Preparation Time:** 5 minutes

**Number of Servings:** 1

**Nutritional Information (per serving):**

- Calories: 250
- Total Fat: 7g
  - Saturated Fat: 0.5g
- Cholesterol: 0mg
- Sodium: 10mg
- Total Carbohydrates: 45g
  - Dietary Fiber: 5g
  - Sugars: 17g
- Protein: 5g

**Chia Seed Pudding**

**Ingredients:**

- 2 tablespoons chia seeds

- 1/2 cup of unsweetened almond milk (or any other non-dairy milk of your choice)
- 1/4 teaspoon vanilla extract
- 1 teaspoon maple syrup (optional)
- Fresh berries for topping

**Preparation:**

- In a bowl or jar, mix together chia seeds, almond milk, vanilla extract, and maple syrup (if using).

- Mix well to combine.

- Cover and refrigerate overnight or for at least 2 hours until the mixture thickens into a pudding-like consistency.

- Serve chilled, topped with fresh berries.

**Preparation Time:** 5 minutes (minus chilling time)

**Number of Servings:** 1

**Nutritional Information (per serving, without toppings):**

- Calories: 120

- Total Fat: 7g
  - Saturated Fat: 0.5g
- Cholesterol: 0mg
- Sodium: 80mg
- Total Carbohydrates: 12g
  - Dietary Fiber: 8g
  - Sugars: 2g
- Protein: 4g

**Spinach and Feta Egg Muffins**

**Ingredients:**

- 4 large eggs
- 1/4 cup chopped spinach
- 1/4 cup crumbled feta cheese
- Salt and pepper to taste
- Non-stick cooking spray

**Preparation:**

- Preheat the oven to 350°F (175°C).

- A muffin tin should be greased with non-stick cooking spray.

- In a mixing bowl, mix the eggs until well combined.

- Add the feta cheese crumbles, chopped spinach, salt, and pepper and stir.

- Pour the egg mixture into the prepared muffin tin, filling each cup about 3/4 full.

- The egg muffins should be baked for 20-25 minutes or until they are set and lightly golden on top.

- Let the egg muffins cool slightly before removing them from the tin.

- Serve warm or refrigerate for later use.

**Cooking Time:** 20-25 minutes

**Number of Servings:** 2

**Nutritional Information (per serving, 2 egg muffins):**

- Calories: 160
- Total Fat: 11g
  - Saturated Fat: 4g
- Cholesterol: 375mg
- Sodium: 280mg
- Total Carbohydrates: 2g
  - Dietary Fiber: 0g

- ○ Sugars: 1g
- Protein: 14g

## Avocado Toast with Tomato and Egg

**Ingredients:**

- 1 slice whole grain or low-FODMAP bread
- 1/4 ripe avocado, mashed
- 1/2 small tomato, sliced
- 1 large egg
- Salt and pepper to taste

**Preparation:**

- Toast the bread until golden brown.

- Lay the mashed avocado evenly on the toast.

- Top with sliced tomato.

- Heat a non-stick skillet over medium heat and cook the egg to your desired doneness (fried, scrambled, or poached).

- Place the cooked egg on top of the avocado and tomato.

- Season with salt and pepper to taste.

- Serve immediately.

**Cooking Time:** 5 minutes

**Number of Servings:** 1

**Nutritional Information (per serving):**

- Calories: 250
- Total Fat: 14g
    - Saturated Fat: 3g
- Cholesterol: 185mg
- Sodium: 170mg
- Total Carbohydrates: 23g
    - Dietary Fiber: 7g
    - Sugars: 3g
- Protein: 11g

**Blueberry Banana Smoothie**

**Ingredients:**

- 1/2 cup frozen blueberries
- 1/2 ripe banana

- 1/2 cup low-fat or non-fat plain Greek yogurt
- 1/2 cup of unsweetened almond milk (or any other non-dairy milk of your choice)
- 1 tablespoon honey (optional)
- 1 tablespoon chia seeds (optional)

**Preparation:**

- Put all the ingredients in a blender.

- Blend until smooth and creamy.

- If desired, taste and adjust sweetness with honey.

- Pour into a glass and sprinkle with chia seeds if using.

- Serve immediately.

**Preparation Time:** 5 minutes

**Number of Servings:** 1

**Nutritional Information (per serving):**

- Calories: 220
- Total Fat: 3g

- ○ Saturated Fat: 0.5g
- Cholesterol: 5mg
- Sodium: 70mg
- Total Carbohydrates: 40g
  - ○ Dietary Fiber: 6g
  - ○ Sugars: 26g
- Protein: 15g

**Peanut Butter Banana Toast**

**Ingredients:**

- 1 slice whole grain or low-FODMAP bread
- 1 tablespoon peanut butter (unsweetened)
- 1/2 ripe banana, sliced
- 1 teaspoon honey (optional)

**Preparation:**

- Toast the bread until golden brown.

- Spread peanut butter evenly on the toast.

- Top with sliced banana.

- If desired, drizzle with honey.

- Serve immediately.

**Preparation Time:** 5 minutes

**Number of Servings:** 1

**Nutritional Information (per serving):**

- Calories: 270
- Total Fat: 11g
    - Saturated Fat: 2g
- Cholesterol: 0mg
- Sodium: 210mg
- Total Carbohydrates: 37g
    - Dietary Fiber: 6g
    - Sugars: 15g
- Protein: 9g

## Almond Butter and Banana Overnight Oats

**Ingredients:**

- 1/2 cup old-fashioned rolled oats
- 1/2 cup of unsweetened almond milk (or any other non-dairy milk of your choice)
- 1 tablespoon almond butter (unsweetened)
- 1/2 ripe banana, mashed

- 1 teaspoon honey (optional)
- 1 tablespoon chopped almonds (optional)

**Preparation:**

- In a jar or container, combine the rolled oats, almond milk, almond butter, mashed banana, and honey (if using).

- Stir well to combine.

- Cover and chill in the refrigerator overnight or for at least 4 hours.

- Before serving, give the oats a stir and top with chopped almonds if desired.

- Serve chilled.

**Preparation Time:** 5 minutes (minus chilling time)

**Number of Servings:** 1

**Nutritional Information (per serving):**

- Calories: 360
- Total Fat: 14g

- ○ Saturated Fat: 1g
- Cholesterol: 0mg
- Sodium: 100mg
- Total Carbohydrates: 50g
  - ○ Dietary Fiber: 8g
  - ○ Sugars: 14g
- Protein: 11g

## Smoked Salmon and Avocado Toast

### Ingredients:

- 1 slice whole grain or low-FODMAP bread
- 1/4 ripe avocado, mashed
- 2 slices smoked salmon
- Fresh dill or chives for garnish (optional)
- Lemon wedges for serving (optional)

### Preparation:

- Toast the bread until golden brown.

- Spread mashed avocado evenly on the toast.

- Arrange smoked salmon slices on top of the avocado.

- Garnish with fresh dill or chives if desired.

- Serve with lemon wedges on the side for squeezing over the toast.

**Preparation Time:** 5 minutes

**Number of Servings:** 1

**Nutritional Information (per serving):**

- Calories: 260
- Total Fat: 13g
    - Saturated Fat: 2g
- Cholesterol: 15mg
- Sodium: 560mg
- Total Carbohydrates: 22g
    - Dietary Fiber: 5g
    - Sugars: 1g
- Protein: 18g

**Vegetable and Egg Breakfast Casserole**

**Ingredients:**

- 4 large eggs
- 1/2 cup diced bell peppers
- 1/2 cup diced tomatoes

- 1/2 cup chopped spinach
- Salt and pepper to taste
- Non-stick cooking spray

**Preparation:**

- Preheat the oven to 350°F (175°C).

- A small baking dish should be greased with non-stick cooking spray.

- In a mixing bowl, mix the eggs until well combined.

- Season with salt and pepper.

- Stir in the diced bell peppers, diced tomatoes, and chopped spinach.

- Transfer the egg mixture into the prepared baking dish.

- Bake the egg mixture for 20-25 minutes or until the eggs are set and the top is lightly golden.

- When slicing and serving, let the casserole cool slightly.

**Cooking Time:** 20-25 minutes

**Number of Servings:** 2

**Nutritional Information (per serving, 1/2 of casserole):**

- Calories: 180
- Total Fat: 10g
    - Saturated Fat: 3g
- Cholesterol: 370mg
- Sodium: 220mg
- Total Carbohydrates: 9g
    - Dietary Fiber: 3g
    - Sugars: 4g
- Protein: 14g

**Coconut Berry Smoothie Bowl**

**Ingredients:**

- 1/2 cup frozen mixed berries (like strawberries, blueberries, raspberries)
- 1/2 ripe banana
- 1/2 cup coconut milk (unsweetened)
- 1 tablespoon unsweetened shredded coconut
- 1 tablespoon chia seeds

- Sliced banana and fresh berries for topping (optional)

## Preparation:

- In a blender, combine the frozen mixed berries, banana, coconut milk, shredded coconut, and chia seeds.

- Blend until smooth and creamy.

- Pour the smoothie into a bowl.

- Top with fresh berries and sliced banana if desired.

- Serve immediately with a spoon.

**Preparation Time:** 5 minutes

**Number of Servings:** 1

**Nutritional Information (per serving):**

- Calories: 310
- Total Fat: 18g
  - Saturated Fat: 14g
- Cholesterol: 0mg
- Sodium: 10mg

- Total Carbohydrates: 36g
  - Dietary Fiber: 9g
  - Sugars: 20g
- Protein: 5g

# Chapter Six

## Pancreatitis-friendly lunch recipes

### Quinoa and Vegetable Salad with Lemon-Tahini Dressing

**Ingredients:**

- 1 cup cooked quinoa
- 1 cup mixed salad greens (like spinach, arugula, and lettuce)
- 1/2 cup diced cucumber
- 1/2 cup diced bell peppers
- 1/4 cup cherry tomatoes, halved
- 1/4 cup diced carrots
- 2 tablespoons chopped fresh parsley
- 2 tablespoons tahini
- 2 tablespoons fresh lemon juice
- 1 tablespoon olive oil
- 1 clove garlic, minced
- Salt and pepper to taste

- Grilled chicken, chickpeas, or tofu for protein (Optional add-ins)

## Preparation:

- In a large mixing bowl, combine the cooked quinoa, mixed salad greens, diced cucumber, diced bell peppers, cherry tomatoes, diced carrots, and chopped fresh parsley.

- In a small bowl, whisk together the tahini, fresh lemon juice, olive oil, minced garlic, salt, and pepper to make the dressing.

- Pour the dressing over the quinoa and vegetable mixture and toss until everything is evenly coated.

- Divide the salad into serving bowls and top with optional add-ins if desired.

- Serve immediately, or refrigerate for later use.

**Preparation Time:** 15 minutes

**Cooking Time:** 15 minutes (for cooking quinoa)

**Number of Servings:** 2

**Nutritional Information (per serving, without optional add-ins):**

- Calories: 300
- Total Fat: 16g
    - Saturated Fat: 2g
- Cholesterol: 0mg
- Sodium: 50mg
- Total Carbohydrates: 32g
    - Dietary Fiber: 5g
    - Sugars: 3g
- Protein: 8g

**Salmon and Avocado Salad**

**Ingredients:**

- 1 can (5 oz) wild-caught salmon, drained
- 1/2 avocado, diced
- 1 cup mixed salad greens (such as spinach, kale, and arugula)
- 1/4 cup cherry tomatoes, halved
- 1/4 cup sliced cucumber

- 1 tablespoon olive oil
- 1 tablespoon lemon juice
- Salt and pepper to taste

**Preparation:**

- In a mixing bowl, combine the drained salmon, diced avocado, mixed salad greens, cherry tomatoes, and sliced cucumber.

- Over the salad, drizzle some lemon juice and olive oil.

- Season with salt and pepper to taste.

- Toss gently to combine.

- Serve immediately.

**Number of Servings: 1**

**Nutritional Information (per serving):**

- Calories: 350
- Total Fat: 24g
    - Saturated Fat: 3.5g
- Cholesterol: 55mg
- Sodium: 250mg

- Total Carbohydrates: 15g
  - Dietary Fiber: 9g
  - Sugars: 3g
- Protein: 24g

**Turkey and Quinoa Stuffed Bell Peppers**

**Ingredients:**

- 2 large bell peppers, halved and seeded
- 1/2 cup cooked quinoa
- 1/2 cup cooked ground turkey (seasoned with salt, pepper, and herbs)
- 1/4 cup diced tomatoes
- 1/4 cup diced zucchini
- 1/4 cup diced onion
- 1/4 cup shredded low-fat mozzarella cheese (optional)
- Salt and pepper to taste
- Olive oil for drizzling

**Preparation:**

- Preheat the oven to 375°F (190°C).

- In a bowl, mix together the cooked quinoa, cooked ground turkey, diced tomatoes, diced zucchini, diced onion, and shredded mozzarella cheese (if using).

- Season with salt and pepper to taste.

- Stuff the halved bell peppers with the quinoa and turkey mixture.

- Lay  the stuffed bell peppers on a baking sheet lined with parchment paper.

- Drizzle with olive oil.

- Bake for 25 to 30 minutes, or until the filling is heated through and the bell peppers are soft.

- Serve hot.

**Cooking Time:** 25-30 minutes

**Number of Servings:** 2

**Nutritional Information (per serving):**

- Calories: 280
- Total Fat: 9g
    - Saturated Fat: 2.5g
- Cholesterol: 40mg

- Sodium: 300mg
- Total Carbohydrates: 26g
  - Dietary Fiber: 6g
  - Sugars: 7g
- Protein: 24g

**Vegetable and Lentil Soup**

**Ingredients:**

- 1/2 cup dry green lentils, rinsed
- 4 cups low-sodium vegetable broth
- 1 cup diced carrots
- 1 cup diced celery
- 1 cup diced zucchini
- 1 cup diced potatoes
- 1/2 cup diced onion
- 2 cloves garlic, minced
- 1 teaspoon dried thyme
- 1 teaspoon dried oregano
- Salt and pepper to taste

**Preparation:**

- In a large pot, combine the rinsed lentils, vegetable broth, diced carrots, diced celery, diced zucchini, diced potatoes, diced onion, minced garlic, dried thyme, and dried oregano.

- Set the heat to medium-high and bring the soup to a boil.

- For 25 to 30 minutes, or until the lentils and vegetables are soft, reduce the heat to low, cover, and simmer.

- Season with salt and pepper to taste.

- Serve hot.

**Cooking Time:** 25-30 minutes

**Number of Servings:** 4

**Nutritional Information (per serving):**

- Calories: 180
- Total Fat: 0.5g
    - Saturated Fat: 0g
- Cholesterol: 0mg
- Sodium: 300mg
- Total Carbohydrates: 33g
    - Dietary Fiber: 10g
    - Sugars: 5g
- Protein: 10g

## Grilled Chicken Salad with Balsamic Vinaigrette

**Ingredients:**

- 2 boneless, skinless chicken breasts
- 4 cups mixed salad greens (like lettuce, spinach, and arugula)
- 1/2 cup cherry tomatoes, halved
- 1/4 cup sliced cucumber
- 1/4 cup sliced red onion
- 1/4 cup sliced avocado
- 2 tablespoons balsamic vinegar
- 1 tablespoon olive oil
- 1 teaspoon Dijon mustard
- Salt and pepper to taste

**Preparation:**

- The grill or grill pan should be preheated over medium-high heat.

- Add salt and pepper to the chicken breasts for seasoning.

- The chicken should be grilled for 6-8 minutes per side or until thoroughly cooked and no longer pink in the middle.

- Take out the chicken from the grill and let it rest for a few minutes before slicing.

- In a large bowl, combine the mixed salad greens, cherry tomatoes, sliced cucumber, sliced red onion, and sliced avocado.

- In a small bowl, mix together the balsamic vinegar, olive oil, Dijon mustard, salt, and pepper to make the dressing.

- Over the salad, drizzle the dressing and toss gently to coat.

- Divide the salad into serving bowls and top with sliced grilled chicken.

- Serve immediately.

**Cooking Time:** 15 minutes

**Number of Servings:** 2

**Nutritional Information (per serving):**

- Calories: 320

- Total Fat: 14g
    - Saturated Fat: 2g
- Cholesterol: 80mg
- Sodium: 200mg
- Total Carbohydrates: 12g
    - Dietary Fiber: 5g
    - Sugars: 4g
- Protein: 34g

**Vegetable Stir-Fry with Tofu**

**Ingredients:**

- 1 cup firm tofu, cubed
- 2 cups mixed stir-fry vegetables (such as bell peppers, broccoli, carrots, and snap peas)
- 2 cloves garlic, minced
- 2 tablespoons low-sodium soy sauce
- 1 tablespoon sesame oil
- 1 teaspoon cornstarch (optional, for thickening sauce)
- Cooked brown rice or quinoa for serving

**Preparation:**

- The sesame oil should be heated in a large skillet or wok over medium-high heat.

- Add minced garlic and cubed tofu to the skillet and cook until tofu is lightly browned on all sides.

- Add mixed stir-fry vegetables to the skillet and stir-fry for 5-7 minutes until vegetables are tender-crisp.

- In a small bowl, mix together soy sauce and cornstarch (if using).

- Turn the soy sauce mixture over the stir-fry and toss to coat.

- Let the sauce thicken by cooking for an additional 2-3 minutes.

- Serve hot on top cooked brown rice or quinoa.

**Cooking Time:** 15 minutes

**Number of Servings:** 2

**Nutritional Information (per serving, without rice/quinoa):**

- Calories: 200

- Total Fat: 10g
  - Saturated Fat: 1.5g
- Cholesterol: 0mg
- Sodium: 500mg
- Total Carbohydrates: 15g
  - Dietary Fiber: 5g
  - Sugars: 5g
- Protein: 15g

**Mediterranean Chickpea Salad**

**Ingredients:**

- 1 can (15 oz) of chickpeas, rinsed and drained
- 1 cup cherry tomatoes, halved
- 1/2 cucumber, diced
- 1/4 cup diced red onion
- 1/4 cup chopped fresh parsley
- 2 tablespoons lemon juice
- 1 tablespoon extra virgin olive oil
- 1 clove garlic, minced
- Salt and pepper to taste
- Crumbled feta cheese (optional)

**Preparation:**

- In a large mixing bowl, add the chickpeas, cherry tomatoes, cucumber, red onion, and chopped parsley.

- In a small bowl, together lemon juice, olive oil, minced garlic, salt, and pepper to make the dressing.

- Pour the dressing over the chickpea salad and toss to coat.

- Add some crumbled feta cheese on top if desired

- Serve chilled or at room temperature.

**Number of Servings:** 4

**Nutritional Information (per serving, without feta cheese):**

- Calories: 180
- Total Fat: 6g
  - Saturated Fat: 0.5g
- Cholesterol: 0mg
- Sodium: 350mg
- Total Carbohydrates: 25g

  - Dietary Fiber: 7g
  - Sugars: 5g
- Protein: 7g

**Turkey and Vegetable Wrap**

**Ingredients:**

- 2 large whole wheat or low-FODMAP tortillas
- 4 slices low-sodium turkey breast
- 1/2 cup mixed salad greens
- 1/4 cup sliced cucumber
- 1/4 cup shredded carrots
- 2 tablespoons hummus
- 1 tablespoon Dijon mustard (optional)

**Preparation:**

- Lay tortillas flat on a clean surface.

- Spread hummus evenly over each tortilla.

- Layer turkey slices, mixed salad greens, sliced cucumber, and shredded carrots on top of the hummus.

- If desired, drizzle with Dijon mustard.

- Fold up the tortillas tightly, folding in the sides to enclose the filling.

- Slice each wrap in half diagonally.

- Serve immediately or wrap tightly in foil for later use.

**Number of Servings:** 2

**Nutritional Information (per serving):**

- Calories: 250
- Total Fat: 6g
  - Saturated Fat: 1g
- Cholesterol: 20mg
- Sodium: 450mg
- Total Carbohydrates: 35g
  - Dietary Fiber: 7g
  - Sugars: 2g
- Protein: 15g

**Caprese Salad with Balsamic Glaze**

**Ingredients:**

- 2 large ripe tomatoes, sliced
- 1 ball fresh mozzarella cheese, sliced

- 1/4 cup fresh basil leaves
- 1 tablespoon balsamic glaze
- 1 tablespoon extra virgin olive oil
- Salt and pepper to taste

## Preparation:

- On a serving platter, arrange alternating slices of tomato and mozzarella cheese.

- Place fresh basil leaves in between the tomato and mozzarella slices.

- Drizzle balsamic glaze and olive oil on top of the salad.

- Season with salt and pepper to taste.

- Serve immediately as a light and refreshing lunch option.

**Number of Servings:** 2

**Nutritional Information (per serving):**

- Calories: 200
- Total Fat: 15g
  - Saturated Fat: 7g
- Cholesterol: 30mg

- Sodium: 300mg
- Total Carbohydrates: 8g
  - Dietary Fiber: 2g
  - Sugars: 4g
- Protein: 10g

**Egg Salad Lettuce Wraps**

**Ingredients:**

- 4 hard-boiled eggs, peeled and chopped
- 2 tablespoons plain Greek yogurt (low-fat or non-fat)
- 1 tablespoon Dijon mustard
- 1 tablespoon chopped fresh dill or chives
- Salt and pepper to taste
- 4 large lettuce leaves (such as butter or romaine)
- Sliced avocado for topping (optional)

**Preparation:**

- In a mixing bowl, combine chopped hard-boiled eggs, Greek yogurt, Dijon mustard, chopped fresh dill or chives, salt, and pepper.

- Mix until well combined.

- Using a spoon, scoop the egg salad mixture onto large lettuce leaves.

- If desired, top with sliced avocado.

- Roll up the lettuce leaves to enclose the filling and form wraps.

- Serve immediately as a light and protein-rich lunch option.

**Number of Servings:** 2

**Nutritional Information (per serving):**

- Calories: 180
- Total Fat: 12g
    - Saturated Fat: 3g
- Cholesterol: 380mg
- Sodium: 260mg
- Total Carbohydrates: 4g
    - Dietary Fiber: 2g
    - Sugars: 1g
- Protein: 14g

**Quinoa Salad with Roasted Vegetables**

**Ingredients:**

- 1 cup cooked quinoa
- 1 cup mixed roasted vegetables (like bell peppers, zucchini, eggplant, and cherry tomatoes)
- 2 tablespoons chopped fresh parsley
- 1 tablespoon extra virgin olive oil
- 1 tablespoon balsamic vinegar
- Salt and pepper to taste

**Preparation:**

- In a large mixing bowl, combine the cooked quinoa and mixed roasted vegetables.

- Add chopped fresh parsley, olive oil, and balsamic vinegar to the bowl.

- Season with salt and pepper to taste.

- Gently toss until all ingredients are thoroughly mixed.

- Serve warm or at room temperature.

**Number of Servings:** 2

**Nutritional Information (per serving):**

- Calories: 220
- Total Fat: 7g
  - Saturated Fat: 1g
- Cholesterol: 0mg
- Sodium: 20mg
- Total Carbohydrates: 35g
  - Dietary Fiber: 5g
  - Sugars: 3g
- Protein: 6g

## Tuna and White Bean Salad

**Ingredients:**

- 1 can (5 oz) of drained tuna in water
- 1 can (15 oz) white beans (like cannellini beans), rinsed and drained
- 1/4 cup diced red onion
- 1/4 cup chopped fresh parsley
- 2 tablespoons lemon juice
- 1 tablespoon extra virgin olive oil
- Salt and pepper to taste
- Cherry tomatoes, sliced cucumber, olives (Optional add-ins)

**Preparation:**

- In a large mixing bowl, add the drained tuna, white beans, diced red onion, and chopped fresh parsley.

- Over the salad, drizzle with olive oil and lemon juice.

- Season with salt and pepper to taste.

- Add optional add-ins if desired.

- Gently toss until all ingredients are thoroughly mixed.

- Serve chilled or at room temperature.

**Number of Servings:** 2

**Nutritional Information (per serving):**

- Calories: 280
- Total Fat: 8g
  - Saturated Fat: 1g
- Cholesterol: 20mg
- Sodium: 460mg
- Total Carbohydrates: 30g

  - ○ Dietary Fiber: 8g
  - ○ Sugars: 1g
- Protein: 24g

## Spinach and Quinoa Stuffed Bell Peppers

### Ingredients:

- 2 large bell peppers, halved and seeded
- 1 cup cooked quinoa
- 1 cup chopped fresh spinach
- 1/2 cup diced tomatoes
- 1/4 cup diced red onion
- 1/4 cup crumbled feta cheese
- 1 tablespoon chopped fresh basil
- Salt and pepper to taste
- Cooked ground turkey, chicken, or tofu (Optional add-ins)

### Preparation:

- Preheat the oven to 375°F (190°C).

- In a large mixing bowl, add cooked quinoa, chopped fresh spinach, diced tomatoes, diced red onion, crumbled feta cheese, chopped fresh basil, salt, and pepper.

- If using optional add-ins, mix them into the quinoa mixture.

- The halved bell peppers should be stuffed with the quinoa mixture.

- Arrange the stuffed bell peppers onto a parchment paper-lined baking sheet.

- Bake the bell peppers for 25-30 minutes or until they are soft.

- Serve hot.

**Cooking Time:** 25-30 minutes

**Number of Servings:** 2

**Nutritional Information (per serving):**

- Calories: 250
- Total Fat: 8g
    - Saturated Fat: 3.5g
- Cholesterol: 20mg
- Sodium: 320mg
- Total Carbohydrates: 35g
    - Dietary Fiber: 7g
    - Sugars: 6g
- Protein: 12g

## Mushroom and Spinach Omelette

**Ingredients:**

- 2 large eggs
- 1/2 cup sliced mushrooms
- 1 cup fresh spinach leaves
- 1/4 cup diced tomatoes
- 2 tablespoons shredded mozzarella cheese
- Salt and pepper to taste
- Cooking spray or olive oil for cooking

**Preparation:**

- In a bowl, mix the eggs until well combined.

- Season with salt and pepper.

- A non-stick skillet should be heated over medium heat and coat with cooking spray or olive oil.

- Add sliced mushrooms to the skillet and cook until softened.

- Add fresh spinach leaves and diced tomatoes to the skillet and cook until spinach is wilted.

- Turn the beaten eggs over the vegetables in the skillet.

- Sprinkle shredded mozzarella cheese on top of the eggs.

- Cook until the omelette is set and the bottom is lightly golden.

- Carefully fold the omelette in half and move to a plate.

- Serve hot.

**Cooking Time:** 10 minutes

**Number of Servings:** 1

**Nutritional Information (per serving):**

- Calories: 270
- Total Fat: 18g
  - Saturated Fat: 6g
- Cholesterol: 380mg
- Sodium: 330mg

- Total Carbohydrates: 8g
  - Dietary Fiber: 2g
  - Sugars: 3g
- Protein: 20g

**Turkey and Avocado Wrap**

**Ingredients:**

- 2 large whole wheat or low-FODMAP tortillas
- 4 slices low-sodium turkey breast
- 1/2 avocado, sliced
- 1/4 cup mixed salad greens
- 2 tablespoons hummus
- Salt and pepper to taste

**Preparation:**

- Lay tortillas flat on a clean surface.

- Spread hummus evenly over each tortilla.

- Layer turkey slices, avocado slices, and mixed salad greens on top of the hummus.

- Season with salt and pepper to taste.

- Fold up the tortillas tightly, folding in the sides to enclose the filling.

- Slice each wrap in half diagonally.

- Serve immediately or wrap tightly in foil for later use.

**Number of Servings:** 2

**Nutritional Information (per serving):**

- Calories: 280
- Total Fat: 12g
  - Saturated Fat: 2g
- Cholesterol: 30mg
- Sodium: 460mg
- Total Carbohydrates: 30g
  - Dietary Fiber: 7g
  - Sugars: 2g
- Protein: 18g

# **Chapter Seven**

## Pancreatitis friendly dinner recipes

**Baked Salmon with Lemon-Dill Sauce**

**Ingredients:**

- 2 salmon fillets (about 6 oz each)
- 1 tablespoon olive oil
- 1 tablespoon fresh lemon juice
- 1 teaspoon lemon zest
- 1 teaspoon dried dill
- Salt and pepper to taste
- Lemon slices for garnish
- For the Lemon-Dill Sauce:
- 1/4 cup plain Greek yogurt (low-fat or non-fat)
- 1 tablespoon fresh lemon juice
- 1 teaspoon lemon zest
- 1 teaspoon dried dill
- Salt and pepper to taste

**Preparation:**

- Preheat the oven to 375°F (190°C).

- Line a baking sheet with parchment paper.

- On the baking sheet that has been prepared, arrange the salmon fillets.

- In a small bowl, mix together olive oil, lemon juice, lemon zest, dried dill, salt, and pepper.

- Coat the salmon fillets evenly by brushing them with the olive oil mixture.

- The salmon should be baked in the preheated oven for 12-15 minutes, or until it's cooked through and flakes easily with a fork.

- While the salmon is baking, make the lemon-dill sauce.

- In a small bowl, mix together Greek yogurt, lemon juice, lemon zest, dried dill, salt, and pepper.

- Once the salmon is cooked, take it out from the oven and let it rest for a few minutes.

- Serve the baked salmon with lemon-dill sauce drizzled on top and garnish with lemon slices.

**Cooking Time:** 12-15 minutes

**Number of Servings:** 2

**Nutritional Information (per serving, without sauce):**

- Calories: 300
- Total Fat: 18g
    - Saturated Fat: 3g
- Cholesterol: 80mg
- Sodium: 70mg
- Total Carbohydrates: 0g
- Protein: 34g

**Nutritional Information (per serving of sauce):**

- Calories: 20
- Total Fat: 0g
- Cholesterol: 0mg
- Sodium: 20mg
- Total Carbohydrates: 1g
- Protein: 3g

**Grilled Chicken Breast with Steamed
Vegetables**

**Ingredients:**

- 2 boneless, skinless chicken breasts
- 1 tablespoon olive oil
- 1 teaspoon dried Italian seasoning
- Salt and pepper to taste
- Assorted steamed vegetables (like broccoli, carrots, and green beans)

**Preparation:**

- The grill or grill pan should be preheated over medium-high heat.

- Brush chicken breasts with olive oil and sprinkle with dried Italian seasoning, salt, and pepper.

- Chicken breasts should be grilled for 6-8 minutes per side or until thoroughly cooked and no longer pink in the middle.

- Serve grilled chicken breasts with steamed vegetables on the side.

**Cooking Time:** 15 minutes

**Number of Servings:** 2

**Nutritional Information (per serving):**

- Calories: 250
- Total Fat: 10g
  - Saturated Fat: 2g
- Cholesterol: 80mg
- Sodium: 150mg
- Total Carbohydrates: 5g
  - Dietary Fiber: 2g
  - Sugars: 2g
- Protein: 35g

**Turkey and Vegetable Stir-Fry**

**Ingredients:**

- 8 oz lean ground turkey
- 2 cups mixed stir-fry vegetables (like bell peppers, broccoli, snap peas, and carrots)
- 2 cloves garlic, minced
- 2 tablespoons low-sodium soy sauce
- 1 tablespoon olive oil
- 1 teaspoon grated ginger
- Salt and pepper to taste

- Cooked brown rice for serving

**Preparation:**

- The olive oil should be heated in a large skillet or wok over medium-high heat.

- Minced garlic and grated ginger should be added to the skillet and cook until fragrant.

- Ground turkey should be added to the skillet and cook until browned and thoroughly cooked.

- Add mixed stir-fry vegetables to the skillet and cook for 5-7 minutes until vegetables are tender-crisp.

- Stir in low-sodium soy sauce and season with salt and pepper to taste.

- Serve turkey and vegetable stir-fry over cooked brown rice.

**Cooking Time:** 15 minutes

**Number of Servings:** 2

**Nutritional Information (per serving, without rice):**

- Calories: 250
- Total Fat: 10g
  - Saturated Fat: 2g
- Cholesterol: 60mg
- Sodium: 400mg
- Total Carbohydrates: 10g
  - Dietary Fiber: 3g
  - Sugars: 4g
- Protein: 30g

**Salmon and Asparagus Foil Packets**

**Ingredients:**

- 2 salmon fillets (about 6 oz each)
- 1 bunch asparagus, trimmed
- 2 tablespoons olive oil
- 2 cloves garlic, minced
- 1 tablespoon lemon juice
- Salt and pepper to taste
- Fresh dill for garnish

**Preparation:**

- Preheat the oven to 375°F (190°C).

- Place each salmon fillet on a piece of aluminum foil large enough to fold into a packet.

- Arrange trimmed asparagus spears around each salmon fillet.

- In a small bowl, add together olive oil, minced garlic, lemon juice, salt, and pepper and mix.

- Over the salmon and asparagus, drizzle the olive oil mixture.

- Fold the aluminum foil over the salmon and asparagus to create packets, sealing tightly.

- Arrange the foil packets on a baking sheet and bake in the preheated oven for 15-20 minutes, or until the salmon is thoroughly cooked.

- Open the foil packets gently and slide the asparagus and salmon onto serving plates.

- Garnish with fresh dill and serve hot.

**Cooking Time:** 15-20 minutes

**Number of Servings:** 2

**Nutritional Information (per serving):**

- Calories: 300
- Total Fat: 20g
  - Saturated Fat: 3g
- Cholesterol: 80mg
- Sodium: 150mg
- Total Carbohydrates: 5g
  - Dietary Fiber: 3g
  - Sugars: 2g
- Protein: 30g

## Quinoa and Black Bean Stuffed Bell Peppers

**Ingredients:**

- 2 big bell peppers, halved and seeded
- 1 cup cooked quinoa
- 1 cup of drained and washed canned black beans
- 1/2 cup diced tomatoes
- 1/4 cup diced red onion
- 1/4 cup shredded cheddar cheese
- 1 teaspoon chili powder

- Salt and pepper to taste
- Fresh cilantro for garnish

**Preparation:**

- Preheat the oven to 375°F (190°C).

- In a large mixing bowl, combine cooked quinoa, black beans, diced tomatoes, diced red onion, shredded cheddar cheese, chili powder, salt, and pepper.

- Using a spoon, scoop the quinoa and black bean mixture into each bell pepper half.

- The stuffed bell peppers should be arranged on a baking sheet lined with parchment paper.

- Bake the stuffed peppers in the preheated oven for 25-30 minutes or until the peppers are soft and the filling is heated through.

- Garnish with fresh cilantro before serving.

**Cooking Time:** 25-30 minutes

**Number of Servings:** 2

**Nutritional Information (per serving):**

- Calories: 300
- Total Fat: 8g
    - Saturated Fat: 3g
- Cholesterol: 15mg
- Sodium: 300mg
- Total Carbohydrates: 45g
    - Dietary Fiber: 10g
    - Sugars: 5g
- Protein: 15g

## Vegetable and Lentil Soup

**Ingredients:**

- 1/2 cup dry green lentils, rinsed
- 4 cups low-sodium vegetable broth
- 1 cup diced carrots
- 1 cup diced celery
- 1 cup diced zucchini
- 1 cup diced potatoes
- 1/2 cup diced onion
- 2 cloves garlic, minced
- 1 teaspoon dried thyme
- 1 teaspoon dried oregano

- Salt and pepper to taste

**Preparation:**

- In a large pot, add the rinsed lentils, low-sodium vegetable broth, diced carrots, celery, zucchini, potatoes, onion, minced garlic, dried thyme, and dried oregano.

- Let the mixture boil over medium-high heat.

- For 25 to 30 minutes, or until the lentils and vegetables are soft, reduce the heat to low, cover, and simmer.

- Season with salt and pepper to taste.

- Serve hot as a comforting and nutritious dinner option.

**Cooking Time:** 25-30 minutes

**Number of Servings:** 4

**Nutritional Information (per serving):**

- Calories: 220

- Total Fat: 1g
- Saturated Fat: 0g
- Cholesterol: 0mg
- Sodium: 250mg
- Total Carbohydrates: 45g
- Dietary Fiber: 15g
- Sugars: 5g
- Protein: 12g

## Roasted Chicken and Vegetable Sheet Pan Dinner

### Ingredients:

- 2 boneless, skinless chicken breasts
- 2 cups mixed vegetables (such as bell peppers, broccoli, cauliflower, and carrots), chopped
- 2 tablespoons olive oil
- 2 cloves garlic, minced
- 1 teaspoon dried thyme
- 1 teaspoon dried rosemary
- Salt and pepper to taste

### Preparation:

- Preheat the oven to 400°F (200°C).

- Line a baking sheet with parchment paper.

- The chicken breasts should be placed in the middle of the baking sheet.

- The mixed vegetables should be arranged around the chicken breasts.

- In a small bowl, mix together olive oil, minced garlic, dried thyme, dried rosemary, salt, and pepper.

- Drizzle the olive oil mixture over the chicken and vegetables, tossing to coat evenly.

- Roast in the preheated oven for 20-25 minutes, or until the chicken is well cooked and the vegetables are soft.

- Serve hot.

**Cooking Time:** 20-25 minutes

**Number of Servings:** 2

**Nutritional Information (per serving):**

- Calories: 300
- Total Fat: 12g
  - Saturated Fat: 2g
- Cholesterol: 80mg
- Sodium: 150mg
- Total Carbohydrates: 15g
  - Dietary Fiber: 5g
  - Sugars: 5g
- Protein: 35g

## Vegetarian Lentil Curry

### Ingredients:

- 1 cup dry green lentils, rinsed
- 2 cups low-sodium vegetable broth
- 1 can (14 oz) diced tomatoes
- 1 can (14 oz) coconut milk
- 1 onion, diced
- 2 cloves garlic, minced
- 1 tablespoon curry powder
- 1 teaspoon ground cumin
- 1 teaspoon ground turmeric
- Salt and pepper to taste
- Fresh cilantro for garnish
- Cooked rice for serving

### Preparation:

- In a large pot, combine the rinsed lentils, low-sodium vegetable broth, diced tomatoes, diced onion, minced garlic, curry powder, ground cumin, ground turmeric, salt, and pepper.

- On medium-high heat, allow the mixture to boil.

- For 25 to 30 minutes, or until the lentils are soft, reduce the heat to low, cover, and simmer.

- Add the coconut milk, stir it and simmer for an additional 5 minutes.

- Garnish with fresh cilantro and serve hot on cooked rice.

**Cooking Time:** 30-35 minutes

**Number of Servings:** 4

**Nutritional Information (per serving, without rice):**

- Calories: 300
- Total Fat: 15g
    - Saturated Fat: 12g

- Cholesterol: 0mg
- Sodium: 300mg
- Total Carbohydrates: 30g
  - Dietary Fiber: 10g
  - Sugars: 5g
- Protein: 15g

**Shrimp and Vegetable Stir-Fry**

**Ingredients:**

- 8 oz shrimp, peeled and deveined
- 2 cups mixed stir-fry vegetables (like bell peppers, snow peas, carrots, and mushrooms)
- 2 cloves garlic, minced
- 2 tablespoons low-sodium soy sauce
- 1 tablespoon olive oil
- 1 teaspoon grated ginger
- 1 teaspoon sesame oil
- Cooked brown rice for serving

**Preparation:**

- The olive oil should be heated in a large skillet or wok over medium-high heat.

- Combine minced garlic and grated ginger to the skillet and cook until fragrant.

- Combine shrimp to the skillet and cook until pink and opaque.

- Add mixed stir-fry vegetables to the skillet and cook for 5-7 minutes until vegetables are tender-crisp.

- Stir in low-sodium soy sauce and sesame oil.

- Serve shrimp and vegetable stir-fry over cooked brown rice.

**Cooking Time:** 10 minutes

**Number of Servings:** 2

**Nutritional Information (per serving, without rice):**

- Calories: 200
- Total Fat: 8g
  - Saturated Fat: 1g
- Cholesterol: 150mg
- Sodium: 350mg

- Total Carbohydrates: 10g
  - Dietary Fiber: 3g
  - Sugars: 4g
- Protein: 20g

**Turkey Meatball Subs**

**Ingredients:**

- 8 turkey meatballs (store-bought or homemade)
- 2 whole wheat or low-FODMAP sub rolls
- 1 cup marinara sauce (store-bought or homemade)
- 1/2 cup shredded mozzarella cheese
- Fresh basil leaves for garnish

**Preparation:**

- Preheat the oven to 375°F (190°C).

- Place turkey meatballs in a baking dish and pour marinara sauce over them.

- The meatballs should be baked in the preheated oven for 15-20 minutes, or until they are thoroughly heated.

- Place the sub rolls on a baking sheet after slicing them in half lengthwise.

- Place 4 meatballs on each sub roll half and sprinkle shredded mozzarella cheese on top.

- Place the baking sheet back in the oven and continue baking for another five minutes, or until the cheese is bubbling and melted.

- Garnish with fresh basil leaves before serving.

**Cooking Time:** 20-25 minutes

**Number of Servings:** 2

**Nutritional Information (per serving):**

- Calories: 350
- Total Fat: 15g
  - Saturated Fat: 5g
- Cholesterol: 80mg
- Sodium: 500mg
- Total Carbohydrates: 30g
  - Dietary Fiber: 5g
  - Sugars: 5g

- Protein: 25g

## Vegetable and Tofu Stir-Fry

## Ingredients:

- 8 oz extra firm tofu, cubed
- 2 cups mixed stir-fry vegetables (like bell peppers, broccoli, snap peas, and carrots)
- 2 cloves garlic, minced
- 2 tablespoons low-sodium soy sauce
- 1 tablespoon olive oil
- 1 teaspoon grated ginger
- Cooked brown rice for serving

## Preparation:

- The olive oil should be heated in a large skillet or wok over medium-high heat.

- Combine minced garlic and grated ginger to the skillet and cook until fragrant.

- Combine cubed tofu to the skillet and cook until lightly browned on all sides.

- Add mixed stir-fry vegetables to the skillet and cook for 5-7 minutes, stirring occasionally, until vegetables are tender-crisp.

- Stir in low-sodium soy sauce and toss to coat evenly.

- Over cooked brown rice, serve the stir-fried vegetables and tofu.

**Cooking Time:** 15 minutes

**Number of Servings:** 2

**Nutritional Information (per serving, without rice):**

- Calories: 250
- Total Fat: 12g
  - Saturated Fat: 2g
- Cholesterol: 0mg
- Sodium: 400mg
- Total Carbohydrates: 20g
  - Dietary Fiber: 5g
  - Sugars: 5g
- Protein: 18g

**Baked Cod with Herbed Quinoa**

**Ingredients:**

- 2 cod fillets (about 6 oz each)
- 1 cup cooked quinoa
- 1 tablespoon olive oil
- 1 tablespoon chopped fresh parsley
- 1 tablespoon chopped fresh dill
- 1 tablespoon lemon juice
- Salt and pepper to taste

**Preparation:**

- Preheat the oven to 375°F (190°C).

- Line a baking sheet with parchment paper.

- Cod fillets should be placed on the prepared baking sheet.

- In a small bowl, mix together cooked quinoa, olive oil, chopped parsley, chopped dill, lemon juice, salt, and pepper.

- Using a spoon, scoop the quinoa mixture over the cod fillets, pressing gently to adhere.

- Bake the cod fillets in the preheated oven for 15-20 minutes, or until they are cooked through and flakes easily with a fork.

- Serve hot.

**Cooking Time:** 15-20 minutes

**Number of Servings:** 2

**Nutritional Information (per serving):**

- Calories: 280
- Total Fat: 9g
  - Saturated Fat: 1g
- Cholesterol: 60mg
- Sodium: 150mg
- Total Carbohydrates: 20g
  - Dietary Fiber: 3g
  - Sugars: 1g
- Protein: 30g

# Chapter Eight

## Pancreatitis-friendly snack recipes

**Greek Yogurt Dip with Veggies**

**Ingredients:**

- 1 cup of low-fat or non-fat plain Greek yogurt
- 1 tablespoon lemon juice
- 1 clove garlic, minced
- 1 tablespoon of fresh or 1 teaspoon of dried dill, chopped
- Salt and pepper to taste
- Assorted vegetables for dipping (carrots, cucumber, bell peppers, celery, etc.)

**Preparation:**

- In a small mixing bowl, add the Greek yogurt, lemon juice, minced garlic, and chopped dill.

- Mix well until smooth.

- Season with salt and pepper to taste, while adjusting as needed.

- To let the flavors melt together, cover the bowl and refrigerate for at least 30 minutes.

- Wash and prepare the assorted vegetables for dipping by cutting them into sticks or slices.

- Serve the Greek yogurt dip with the prepared vegetables.

**Preparation time:** (10 minutes + 30 minutes chilling)

**Number of Servings:** 4

**Nutritional Information (per serving, including dip and vegetables):**

- Calories: 70
- Fat: 0.5g
- Carbohydrates: 8g
- Fiber: 2g
- Protein: 8g

## Avocado and Tomato Salad

### Ingredients:

- 1 ripe avocado, diced
- 1 tomato, diced
- 1 tablespoon fresh cilantro, chopped
- 1 tablespoon lime juice
- Salt and pepper to taste

### Preparation:

- In a bowl, combine the diced avocado, tomato, and chopped cilantro.

- Drizzle lime juice over the mixture and gently toss to mix.

- Season with salt and pepper to taste.

- Serve right away or chill in the refrigerator until you are ready to eat.

**Number of Servings:** 2

**Nutritional Information (per serving):**

- Calories: 120
- Fat: 10g

- Carbohydrates: 7g
- Fiber: 5g
- Protein: 2g

## Apple and Almond Butter Slices

## Ingredients:

- 1 apple, sliced
- 2 tablespoons almond butter (or any nut butter of choice)
- Cinnamon (optional)

## Preparation:

- Slice the apple into thin rounds or wedges, removing the core.

- Spread almond butter on each apple slice.

- Sprinkle with cinnamon if desired.

- Arrange on a plate and serve immediately.

## Number of Servings: 2

**Nutritional Information (per serving):**

- Calories: 150
- Fat: 9g
- Carbohydrates: 18g
- Fiber: 4g
- Protein: 3g

**Rice Cake with Cottage Cheese and Berries**

**Ingredients:**

- 2 rice cakes (plain or lightly salted)
- 1/4 cup low-fat cottage cheese
- 1/4 cup mixed berries (strawberries, blueberries, raspberries)

**Preparation:**

- Spread cottage cheese evenly on each rice cake.

- Top with mixed berries.

- Serve immediately.

**Number of Servings:** 2

**Nutritional Information (per serving):**

- Calories: 100
- Fat: 1g
- Carbohydrates: 18g
- Fiber: 2g
- Protein: 5g

**Hummus and Veggie Sticks**

**Ingredients:**

- 1/2 cup hummus (store-bought or homemade)
- Assorted vegetable sticks (carrots, cucumbers, bell peppers, celery)

**Preparation:**

- In a small bowl, hummus should be placed for dipping.

- Wash and cut the vegetables into sticks.

- Arrange the vegetable sticks around the bowl of hummus on a serving platter.

- Serve immediately.

**Number of Servings:** 2

**Nutritional Information (per serving, including hummus and vegetables):**

- Calories: 120
- Fat: 6g
- Carbohydrates: 13g
- Fiber: 6g
- Protein: 5g

**Almond Butter Banana Bites**

**Ingredients:**

- 1 banana, peeled and sliced
- 2 tablespoons almond butter (or any nut butter of choice)
- Unsweetened shredded coconut (optional)

**Preparation:**

- Spread almond butter on each banana slice.

- Roll each almond butter-coated banana slice in shredded coconut for added flavor and texture (Optional).

- Arrange on a plate and eat immediately.

**Number of Servings:** 2

**Nutritional Information (per serving):**

- Calories: 160
- Fat: 9g
- Carbohydrates: 20g
- Fiber: 3g
- Protein: 4g

## Cottage Cheese and Pineapple Spears

**Ingredients:**

- 1/2 cup low-fat cottage cheese
- 1 cup fresh pineapple, cut into spears

**Preparation:**

- Place the cottage cheese in a small bowl for dipping.

- Serve alongside fresh pineapple spears.

**Number of Servings:** 2

**Nutritional Information (per serving, including cottage cheese and pineapple):**

- Calories: 120
- Fat: 1g
- Carbohydrates: 20g
- Fiber: 2g
- Protein: 8g

**Tuna Salad Lettuce Wraps**

**Ingredients:**

- 1 can (5 oz) tuna, drained
- 2 tablespoons plain Greek yogurt
- 1 tablespoon lemon juice
- 1 tablespoon chopped celery
- Salt and pepper to taste
- Lettuce leaves for wrapping

**Preparation:**

- In a bowl, combine the drained tuna, Greek yogurt, lemon juice, chopped celery, salt, and pepper.

- Mix until well combined.

- Spoon the tuna salad onto lettuce leaves.

- Fold up the lettuce leaves to form wraps.

- Serve immediately.

**Number of Servings:** 2

**Nutritional Information (per serving):**

- Calories: 110
- Fat: 2g
- Carbohydrates: 2g
- Fiber: 0g
- Protein: 20g

**Egg Salad Cucumber Bites**

**Ingredients:**

- 2 hard-boiled eggs, chopped
- 1 tablespoon plain Greek yogurt
- 1 teaspoon Dijon mustard
- Salt and pepper to taste
- 1 cucumber, sliced into rounds

## Preparation:

- In a bowl, combine the chopped hard-boiled eggs, Greek yogurt, Dijon mustard, salt, and pepper.

- Mix until well combined.

- Spoon the egg salad onto cucumber slices.

- Serve immediately.

**Number of Servings: 2**

**Nutritional Information (per serving):**

- Calories: 100
- Fat: 6g
- Carbohydrates: 4g
- Fiber: 1g
- Protein: 8g

## Turkey and Cheese Roll-Ups

**Ingredients:**

- 4 slices deli turkey breast

- 2 slices low-fat cheese (such as Swiss or cheddar)
- Mustard or hummus for spreading (optional)

**Preparation:**

- Arrange the turkey slices on a clean surface.

- Top each turkey slice with a slice of cheese.

- Spread a thin layer of mustard or hummus on top of the cheese (Optional).

- Roll up each turkey slice into a tight cylinder.

- Secure with toothpicks if needed.

- Serve right away or chill in the refrigerator until you are ready to eat.

**Number of Servings:** 2

**Nutritional Information (per serving, including 2 roll-ups):**

- Calories: 180
- Fat: 9g
- Carbohydrates: 2g
- Fiber: 0g
- Protein: 20g

# Chapter Nine

## Pancreatitis-friendly side dish recipes

### Steamed Vegetables with Lemon Herb Dressing

**Ingredients:**

- Assorted vegetables (broccoli, cauliflower, carrots, and zucchini), washed and chopped into bite-sized pieces
- 1 tablespoon olive oil
- 1 tablespoon lemon juice
- 1 teaspoon fresh or 1/2 teaspoon dried thyme, chopped
- Salt and pepper to taste

**Preparation:**

- Place the chopped vegetables in a steamer basket over boiling water.

- Steam the vegetables for 5-7 minutes or until they are tender but still crisp.

- While the vegetables are steaming, prepare the dressing by whisking together olive oil, lemon juice, chopped thyme, salt, and pepper in a small bowl.

- Once the vegetables are done, transfer them to a serving dish and drizzle the lemon herb dressing over the top.

- Mix gently to coat the vegetables evenly with the dressing.

- Serve hot as a side dish.

**Number of Servings:** 4

**Nutritional Information (per serving):**

- Calories: 70
- Fat: 4g
- Carbohydrates: 8g
- Fiber: 3g
- Protein: 2g

## Quinoa and Vegetable Stir-Fry

**Ingredients:**

- 1 cup quinoa, rinsed
- 2 cups water or low-sodium vegetable broth
- 1 tablespoon olive oil
- 2 cloves garlic, minced
- 1 small onion, diced
- 2 cups mixed vegetables (bell peppers, snap peas, carrots, and broccoli), chopped
- 2 tablespoons low-sodium soy sauce
- 1 tablespoon rice vinegar
- 1 teaspoon sesame oil
- 1/4 cup chopped green onions (optional)
- Sesame seeds for garnish (optional)

**Preparation:**

- In a medium saucepan, add the quinoa and water or vegetable broth.

- Let it boil, then for 15-20 minutes reduce heat to low, cover and simmer or until the quinoa is cooked and liquid is absorbed.

- Take out from the heat, cover, and let settle for five minutes before fluffing with a fork..

- The olive oil should be heated in a large skillet or wok, over medium heat.

- Add minced garlic and diced onion, and sauté for 2-3 minutes until softened.

- Combine the chopped mixed vegetables to the skillet and stir-fry for 5-7 minutes or until they are soft but still crisp.

- Mix together soy sauce, rice vinegar, and sesame oil in a small bowl.

- Add the cooked quinoa to the skillet with the vegetables and pour the sauce over the top.

- Stir to combine and heat through.

- Take out from heat and if desired, garnish with chopped green onions and sesame seeds.

- Serve hot as a side dish.

**Number of Servings:** 4

**Nutritional Information (per serving):**

- Calories: 220
- Fat: 7g
- Carbohydrates: 33g
- Fiber: 5g
- Protein: 7g

**Mashed Sweet Potatoes**

**Ingredients:**

- 2 medium sweet potatoes, peeled and diced
- 2 tablespoons of unsalted butter (or olive oil for a dairy-free option)
- 1/4 cup of low-fat milk (or unsweetened almond milk for a dairy-free option)
- Salt and pepper to taste
- Chopped chives for garnish (optional)

**Preparation:**

- The diced sweet potatoes should be put into a large saucepan and cover with water.

- Bring to a boil over medium-high heat, then reduce the heat to low and simmer for 15-20 minutes or until the sweet potatoes are fork-tender.

- After draining the sweet potatoes, transfer them to a mixing bowl.

- Add butter (or olive oil) and milk to the sweet potatoes.

- Mash the sweet potatoes using a potato masher until smooth and creamy.

- If additional milk is needed to get the right consistency, add it.

- Season with salt and pepper to taste.

- Garnish with chopped chives if desired before serving.

**Number of Servings: 4**

**Nutritional Information (per serving):**

- Calories: 130
- Fat: 4g
- Carbohydrates: 22g

- Fiber: 3g
- Protein: 2g

## Roasted Brussels Sprouts

### Ingredients:

- 1 pound Brussels sprouts, trimmed and halved
- 2 tablespoons olive oil
- 2 cloves garlic, minced
- Salt and pepper to taste
- Grated Parmesan cheese for serving (optional)

### Preparation:

- Preheat your oven to 400°F (200°C).

- In a large bowl, mix the Brussels sprouts with olive oil, minced garlic, salt, and pepper until evenly coated.

- Lay the Brussels sprouts in a single layer on a baking sheet lined with parchment paper.

- Roast in the preheated oven for 20-25 minutes, stirring halfway through, or until the Brussels sprouts are tender and caramelized.

- Take out from the oven and transfer to a serving dish.

- Sprinkle with grated Parmesan cheese if desired before serving.

**Number of Servings:** 4

**Nutritional Information (per serving):**

- Calories: 90
- Fat: 7g
- Carbohydrates: 7g
- Fiber: 3g
- Protein: 3g

**Quinoa and Black Bean Salad**

**Ingredients:**

- 1 cup quinoa, rinsed
- 2 cups water or low-sodium vegetable broth
- 1 can (15 oz) of rinsed and drained black beans
- 1 bell pepper, diced

- 1/4 cup red onion, finely chopped
- 1/4 cup fresh cilantro, chopped
- 2 tablespoons olive oil
- 2 tablespoons lime juice
- Salt and pepper to taste
- Avocado slices for garnish (optional)

**Preparation:**

- In a medium saucepan, add the quinoa and water or vegetable broth.

- Allow it to boil, then for 15-20 minutes, reduce the heat to low, cover and simmer or until the quinoa is cooked and liquid is absorbed.

- Take out from heat and let it cool.

- In a large mixing bowl, add the cooked quinoa, black beans, diced bell pepper, chopped red onion, and chopped cilantro and mix

- In a small bowl, whisk together olive oil, lime juice, salt, and pepper.

- Turn the dressing over the quinoa mixture and mix until everything is well coated.

- Adjust seasoning if needed and garnish with avocado slices before serving.

**Number of Servings:** 4

**Nutritional Information (per serving):**

- Calories: 280
- Fat: 9g
- Carbohydrates: 40g
- Fiber: 9g
- Protein: 11g

**Baked Acorn Squash**

**Ingredients:**

- 2 acorn squash, halved and seeds removed
- 2 tablespoons of unsalted butter (or olive oil for a dairy-free option)
- 2 tablespoons maple syrup (optional)
- Salt and pepper to taste
- Cinnamon for sprinkling (optional)

**Preparation:**

- Preheat your oven to 400°F (200°C).

- The halved acorn squash should be placed on a baking sheet, cut side up.

- Place a small pat of butter (or drizzle olive oil) inside each squash half.

- If using maple syrup, drizzle it over the squash halves.

- Season with salt, pepper, and a sprinkle of cinnamon if desired.

- Roast the squash in the preheated oven for 40-45 minutes or until the squash is soft and caramelized.

- Take out from the oven and before serving, let it cool slightly.

**Number of Servings:** 4

**Nutritional Information (per serving):**

- Calories: 120
- Fat: 5g

- Carbohydrates: 22g
- Fiber: 3g
- Protein: 2g

**Cucumber and Tomato Salad**

**Ingredients:**

- 2 cucumbers, diced
- 2 tomatoes, diced
- 1/4 cup red onion, finely chopped
- 2 tablespoons fresh parsley, chopped
- 2 tablespoons olive oil
- 1 tablespoon lemon juice
- Salt and pepper to taste

**Preparation:**

- In a large bowl, add the diced cucumbers, tomatoes, red onion, and parsley.

- In a small bowl, mix together the olive oil, lemon juice, salt, and pepper to make the dressing.

- Turn the dressing over the cucumber and tomato mixture and mix until evenly coated.

- If necessary, adjust the seasoning, and chill in the refrigerator for at least half an hour before serving.

**Number of Servings:** 4

**Nutritional Information (per serving):**

- Calories: 80
- Fat: 7g
- Carbohydrates: 5g
- Fiber: 1g
- Protein: 1g

**Oven-Roasted Asparagus**

**Ingredients:**

- 1 bunch asparagus, woody ends trimmed
- 1 tablespoon olive oil
- Salt and pepper to taste
- Lemon wedges for serving (optional)

**Preparation:**

- Preheat your oven to 400°F (200°C).

- Lay the trimmed asparagus spears on a baking sheet lined with parchment paper.

- Over the asparagus, drizzle olive oil and mix to coat evenly.

- Season with salt and pepper to taste.

- Roast the asparagus in the preheated oven for 12-15 minutes, or until the asparagus is soft and slightly browned.

- Take out from the oven and serve with lemon wedges if desired.

**Number of Servings:** 4

**Nutritional Information (per serving):**

- Calories: 40
- Fat: 3g
- Carbohydrates: 3g
- Fiber: 2g
- Protein: 2g

**Baked Butternut Squash Fries**

**Ingredients:**

- 1 medium of peeled and seeded butternut squash cut into fries
- 1 tablespoon olive oil
- 1/2 teaspoon garlic powder
- 1/2 teaspoon paprika
- Salt and pepper to taste

**Preparation:**

- Preheat your oven to 425°F (220°C).

- In a large bowl, toss the butternut squash fries with olive oil, garlic powder, paprika, salt, and pepper until evenly coated.

- The fries should be arranged in a single layer on a baking sheet lined with parchment paper.

- Bake in the preheated oven for 20-25 minutes, flipping halfway through, or until the fries are golden brown and crispy.

- Remove from the oven and serve hot.

**Number of Servings:** 4

**Nutritional Information (per serving):**

- Calories: 70
- Fat: 3g
- Carbohydrates: 12g
- Fiber: 3g
- Protein: 1g

**Sauteed Spinach with Garlic**

**Ingredients:**

- 1 tablespoon olive oil
- 2 cloves garlic, minced
- 8 cups fresh spinach leaves
- Salt and pepper to taste
- Lemon wedges for serving (optional)

**Preparation:**

- The olive oil should be heated in a large skillet over medium heat.

- Toss the minced garlic to the skillet and sauté for 1-2 minutes until fragrant.

- Add fresh spinach leaves to the skillet in batches, tossing gently until wilted.

- Season with salt and pepper to taste.

- Take out from heat and serve immediately with lemon wedges if desired.

**Number of Servings:** 4

**Nutritional Information (per serving):**

- Calories: 40
- Fat: 3g
- Carbohydrates: 3g
- Fiber: 2g
- Protein: 2g

# Chapter Ten

## Pancreatitis-friendly dessert recipes

**Baked Apples**

**Ingredients:**

- 4 apples (like Granny Smith or Honeycrisp), cored
- 2 tablespoons unsalted butter (or coconut oil for a dairy-free option)
- 2 tablespoons honey (optional)
- 1 teaspoon ground cinnamon
- 1/4 cup chopped nuts (walnuts or pecans)

**Preparation:**

- Preheat your oven to 375°F (190°C).

- The cored apples should be placed in a baking dish.

- The butter (or coconut oil) should be melted in a small saucepan over low heat.

- Stir in honey (if using) and cinnamon until well combined.

- Pour the butter mixture over the apples, making sure to coat each one evenly.

- Over the top of each Apple, sprinkle chopped nuts.

- Bake the apples in the preheated oven for 25-30 minutes or until they  are soft.

- Take out from the oven and let cool slightly before serving.

**Number of Servings:** 4

**Nutritional Information (per serving):**

- Calories: 150
- Fat: 7g
- Carbohydrates: 24g
- Fiber: 5g
- Protein: 1g

## Banana "Nice" Cream

**Ingredients:**

- 2 ripe bananas, peeled and sliced
- 1/4 cup of unsweetened almond milk (or any other milk of your choice)
- 1 teaspoon vanilla extract (optional)
- Toppings of choice (chopped nuts, berries, or shredded coconut)

**Preparation:**

- The sliced bananas should be arranged on a baking sheet lined with parchment paper.

- For 2 hours freeze the banana slices or until they are completely frozen.

- Once frozen, the banana slices should be transferred to a blender or food processor.

- Add almond milk and vanilla extract (if using) to the blender.

- Blend, scraping down the sides as needed, until creamy and smooth.

- For a firmer texture, transfer to a container and freeze, or serve immediately as soft-serve ice cream.

- Top with your favorite toppings before serving.

**Number of Servings:** 2

**Nutritional Information (per serving, without toppings):**

- Calories: 100
- Fat: 1g
- Carbohydrates: 25g
- Fiber: 3g
- Protein: 1g

**Greek Yogurt Parfait**

**Ingredients:**

- 1 cup of low-fat or non-fat plain Greek yoghourt
- 1/4 cup granola (choose a low-sugar option)
- 1/2 cup mixed berries (strawberries, blueberries, raspberries)

- Honey or maple syrup for drizzling (optional)

**Preparation:**

- Layer Greek yogurt, granola, and mixed berries in a serving bowl or glass.

- Repeat layering until the serving bowl or glass is filled.

- If desired, drizzle honey or maple syrup on the top.

- Serve immediately as a delicious and nutritious dessert or snack.

**Number of Servings:** 1

**Nutritional Information (per serving):**

- Calories: 250
- Fat: 5g
- Carbohydrates: 35g
- Fiber: 5g
- Protein: 20g

## Rice Pudding

### Ingredients:

- 1 cup cooked white rice (short-grain or long-grain)
- 1 cup of low-fat milk
- 2 tablespoons honey (or maple syrup)
- 1/2 teaspoon ground cinnamon
- 1/2 teaspoon vanilla extract
- Raisins or chopped nuts for garnish (optional)

### Preparation:

- In a saucepan, combine cooked rice, milk, honey, cinnamon, and vanilla extract.

- Cook over medium heat, stirring frequently, until the mixture thickens and reaches your desired consistency (about 10-15 minutes).

- Take out from heat and let cool slightly.

- Serve warm or chilled, garnished with raisins or chopped nuts if desired.

**Number of Servings:** 2

**Nutritional Information (per serving, without garnishes):**

- Calories: 250
- Fat: 2g
- Carbohydrates: 55g
- Fiber: 1g
- Protein: 6g

**Berry Chia Seed Pudding**

**Ingredients:**

- 1/4 cup chia seeds
- 1 cup of unsweetened almond milk (or any other type of milk of your choice)
- 1 tablespoon honey (or maple syrup)
- 1/2 teaspoon vanilla extract
- 1/2 cup mixed berries (strawberries, blueberries, raspberries)

**Preparation:**

- In a bowl, add chia seeds, almond milk, honey, and vanilla extract. Stir well to combine.

- For at least 2 hours or overnight, cover the bowl and store in the refrigerator allowing the chia seeds to absorb the liquid and thicken.

- Stir the pudding mixture before serving to ensure even consistency.

- Serve topped with mixed berries.

**Number of Servings:** 2

**Nutritional Information (per serving):**

- Calories: 180
- Fat: 8g
- Carbohydrates: 24g
- Fiber: 12g
- Protein: 5g

**Frozen Banana Bites**

**Ingredients:**

- 2 ripe bananas, peeled and sliced into rounds
- 1/4 cup of unsweetened almond butter (or any nut butter of your choice)

- 1/4 cup dark chocolate chips (minimum 70% cocoa)
- 1 tablespoon coconut oil
- For coating, chopped nuts or shredded coconut (optional).

**Preparation:**

- Arrange banana slices on a parchment-lined baking sheet.

- Spread almond butter on half of the banana slices and top with the remaining slices to create sandwiches.

- Insert a toothpick into each banana sandwich and place the baking sheet in the freezer for at least 1 hour to firm up.

- Melt dark chocolate chips and coconut oil in a microwave-safe bowl, in 30-second intervals, stirring until smooth.

- Dip each frozen banana sandwich into the melted chocolate to coat evenly.

- Roll the chocolate-coated bananas in chopped nuts or shredded coconut (Optional).

- Return the coated banana bites to the baking sheet and freeze for an additional 30 minutes or until the chocolate sets.

- Serve chilled as a delicious frozen treat.

**Number of Servings:** 4

**Nutritional Information (per serving):**

- Calories: 160
- Fat: 10g
- Carbohydrates: 18g
- Fiber: 3g
- Protein: 3g

**Coconut Mango Sorbet**

**Ingredients:**

- 2 cups frozen mango chunks
- 1/2 cup canned coconut milk (light or full-fat)
- 2 tablespoons honey (or maple syrup)

- 1 tablespoon lime juice

**Preparation:**

- In a blender or food processor, add frozen mango chunks, coconut milk, honey, and lime juice.

- Blend, scraping down the sides as needed, until creamy and smooth.

- If necessary, taste and adjust sweetness by adding more honey or maple syrup.

- Serve immediately as soft-serve sorbet or transfer to a container and freeze for a firmer texture.

- If desired, before serving, garnish with fresh mint leaves or shredded coconut.

**Number of Servings:** 4

**Nutritional Information (per serving):**

- Calories: 150
- Fat: 6g
- Carbohydrates: 26g
- Fiber: 2g

- Protein: 1g

## Oatmeal Raisin Cookies

**Ingredients:**

- 1 cup rolled oats
- 1/2 cup whole wheat flour
- 1/4 cup unsweetened applesauce
- 1/4 cup honey (or maple syrup)
- 1/4 cup raisins
- 1/2 teaspoon ground cinnamon
- 1/4 teaspoon baking soda
- 1/4 teaspoon salt

**Preparation:**

- Preheat your oven to 350°F (175°C).

- Line a baking sheet with parchment paper.

- In a large bowl, add rolled oats, whole wheat flour, cinnamon, baking soda, and salt.

- Stir in unsweetened applesauce, honey, and raisins until well combined and a dough forms.

- Spacing them apart, drop spoonfuls of dough onto the prepared baking sheet.

- With the back of a spoon or your fingers, flatten each cookie slightly.

- Bake the cookies in the preheated oven for 10-12 minutes or until the cookies are golden brown.

- Take out from the oven and let it cool on the baking sheet for 5 minutes before transferring to a wire rack to cool completely.

**Number of Servings:** 12

**Nutritional Information (per serving, based on 1 cookie):**

- Calories: 90
- Fat: 1g
- Carbohydrates: 19g
- Fiber: 2g
- Protein: 2g

## Pumpkin Spice Smoothie

**Ingredients:**

- 1/2 cup canned pumpkin puree
- 1 ripe banana
- 1/2 cup unsweetened almond milk (or any milk of choice)
- 1/4 teaspoon ground cinnamon
- 1/4 teaspoon ground nutmeg
- 1/4 teaspoon ground ginger
- 1/4 teaspoon vanilla extract
- 1 tablespoon honey (or maple syrup)
- Ice cubes (optional)

**Preparation:**

- In a blender, add pumpkin puree, banana, almond milk, cinnamon, nutmeg, ginger, vanilla extract, and honey.

- If desired, add ice cubes for a colder consistency.

- Blend until smooth and creamy.

- Pour into glasses and serve immediately, optionally garnished with a sprinkle of cinnamon on top.

**Number of Servings:** 2

**Nutritional Information (per serving):**

- Calories: 120
- Fat: 1g
- Carbohydrates: 28g
- Fiber: 5g
- Protein: 2g

**Lemon Blueberry Frozen Yogurt**

**Ingredients:**

- 2 cups of low-fat or non-fat  plain Greek yogurt
- 1 cup frozen blueberries
- 1/4 cup honey (or maple syrup)
- Zest and juice of 1 lemon

**Preparation:**

- In a blender or food processor, add Greek yogurt, frozen blueberries, honey, lemon zest, and lemon juice.

- Blend, scraping down the sides as needed, until creamy and smooth.

- If necessary, taste and adjust sweetness by adding more honey.

- Serve immediately as soft-serve frozen yogurt or transfer to a container and freeze for a firmer texture.

- If desired, before serving, garnish with fresh blueberries and lemon zest.

**Number of Servings:** 4

**Nutritional Information (per serving):**

- Calories: 140
- Fat: 0g
- Carbohydrates: 28g
- Fiber: 2g
- Protein: 7g

# Chapter Eleven

## 4 weeks meal plan

Week One

**Day 1:**

**Breakfast:**

- Oatmeal with sliced banana and honey drizzled on top.
- Herbal tea or water.

**Lunch:**

- Quinoa, steamed broccoli, and grilled chicken breast.
- Mixed green salad with olive oil and lemon dressing.

**Dinner:**

- Sautéed spinach and roasted sweet potatoes with baked salmon

- Sliced cucumber and tomato salad with balsamic vinaigrette.

**Snack:**

- Greek yogurt with mixed berries.

**Day 2:**

**Breakfast:**

- Scrambled eggs with spinach and tomatoes.
- Whole grain toast with almond butter.
- Herbal tea or water.

**Lunch:**

- Whole wheat tortilla wrapped with turkey and avocado.
- Carrot sticks with hummus.

**Dinner:**

- Whole grain bread on the side with lentil soup.
- Mixed green salad with olive oil and vinegar dressing.

**Snack:**

- Apple slices with a sprinkle of cinnamon.

**Day 3:**

**Breakfast:**

- Greek yogurt parfait topped with mixed berries and granola.
- Herbal tea or water.

**Lunch:**

- Grilled shrimp and mixed veggies with quinoa salad.
- Sliced bell peppers with tzatziki sauce.

**Dinner:**

- Roasted Brussels sprouts, brown rice, and baked chicken thighs.
- Steamed asparagus with lemon zest.

**Snack:**

- Cottage cheese with pineapple chunks.

**Day 4:**

**Breakfast:**

- Poached eggs and mashed avocado with whole grain bread.
- Herbal tea or water.

**Lunch:**

- Tuna salad lettuce wraps with cucumber slices.
- Handful of almonds.

**Dinner:**

- Brown rice, broccoli, and bell peppers stir-fried with tofu.
- Mixed green salad with lemon-tahini dressing.

**Snack:**

- Strawberry slices and almond butter on a rice cake.

**Day 5:**

**Breakfast:**

- Spinach, banana, almond milk, and a scoop of protein powder smoothie.
- Herbal tea or water.

**Lunch:**

- Quinoa and black bean salad with diced tomatoes and avocado.
- Carrot sticks with hummus.

**Dinner:**

- Steamed green beans and quinoa pilaf with baked cod.
- Sliced cucumber and tomato salad with balsamic vinaigrette.

**Snack:**

- Cottage cheese with sliced peaches.

**Day 6:**

**Breakfast:**

- Chia seeds, almond milk, and mixed berries with overnight oats.
- Herbal tea or water.

**Lunch:**

- Chicken and vegetable stir-fry with brown rice.
- Sliced bell peppers with hummus.

**Dinner:**

- Turkey meatballs with marinara sauce over spaghetti squash noodles.
- Mixed green salad with olive oil and lemon dressing.

**Snack:**

- Greek yogurt with honey and chopped nuts.

**Day 7:**

**Breakfast:**

- Whole grain toast with scrambled eggs and sliced avocado.
- Herbal tea or water.

**Lunch:**

- Vegetable and lentil soup with wholegrain bread.
- Carrot sticks with tzatziki sauce.

**Dinner:**

- Steamed broccoli and roasted sweet potatoes served with grilled shrimp skewers.
- Mixed green salad with balsamic vinaigrette.

**Snack:**

- Apple slices with almond butter.

## Week Two

**Day 1:**

**Breakfast:**

- Smoothie made with banana, spinach, unsweetened almond milk, and a scoop of protein powder.
- Herbal tea or water.

**Lunch:**

- Grilled chicken salad with mixed greens, cherry tomatoes, cucumber, and balsamic vinaigrette.
- Whole grain roll.

**Dinner:**

- Baked tilapia with quinoa pilaf and steamed asparagus.
- Sliced bell peppers with hummus.

**Snack:**

- Greek yogurt with a drizzle of honey.

**Day 2:**

**Breakfast:**

- Almond milk, chia seeds, rolled oats, and sliced strawberries combine to make overnight oats.
- Herbal tea or water.

**Lunch:**

- Whole wheat tortilla with turkey and avocado wrap.
- Carrot sticks with tzatziki sauce.

**Dinner:**

- Vegetable stir-fry with tofu, bell peppers, broccoli, and snap peas served over brown rice.
- Mixed green salad with lemon-tahini dressing.

**Snack:**

- Apple slices with almond butter.

**Day 3:**

**Breakfast:**

- Scrambled eggs with sautéed spinach and tomatoes.
- Whole grain toast with mashed avocado.
- Herbal tea or water.

**Lunch:**

- Quinoa and black bean salad topped with diced avocado and lime dressing
- Handful of mixed nuts.

**Dinner:**

- Baked salmon with roasted sweet potatoes and green beans.
- Mixed green salad with balsamic vinaigrette.

**Snack:**

- Cottage cheese with pineapple chunks.

**Day 4:**

## Breakfast:

- Greek yogurt parfait topped with mixed berries and granola.
- Herbal tea or water.

## Lunch:

- Whole grain bread on the side with lentil soup.
- Sliced cucumber with hummus.

## Dinner:

- Chicken and vegetable kebabs with quinoa and steamed broccoli.
- Mixed green salad with lemon-tahini dressing.

## Snack:

- Banana slices with almond butter on a rice cake.

**Day 5:**

**Breakfast:**

- Whole grain toast with scrambled eggs and sliced avocado.
- Herbal tea or water.

**Lunch:**

- Tuna salad lettuce wraps with cucumber slices.
- Carrot sticks with hummus.

**Dinner:**

- Roasted brussels sprouts and quinoa pilaf served with baked cod.
- Mixed green salad with balsamic vinaigrette.

**Snack:**

- Greek yogurt with honey and chopped nuts.

**Day 6:**

**Breakfast:**

- Smoothie made with mixed berries, spinach, unsweetened almond milk, and a scoop of protein powder.
- Herbal tea or water.

**Lunch:**

- Grilled shrimp salad with mixed greens, cherry tomatoes, cucumber, and lemon-tahini dressing.
- Whole grain roll.

**Dinner:**

- Turkey meatballs with marinara sauce over spaghetti squash noodles.
- Mixed green salad with balsamic vinaigrette.

**Snack:**

- Apple slices with almond butter.

**Day 7:**

**Breakfast:**

- Oatmeal with sliced banana and honey drizzled on top.
- Herbal tea or water.

**Lunch:**

- Chickpea salad with mixed greens, diced bell peppers, cherry tomatoes, and lemon-tahini dressing.
- Handful of mixed nuts.

**Dinner:**

- Baked chicken breast with quinoa and steamed green beans.
- Mixed green salad with balsamic vinaigrette.

**Snack:**

- Cottage cheese with sliced peaches.

## Week Three

### Day 1:

### Breakfast:

- scrambled eggs with spinach and chopped bell peppers.
- Whole grain toast topped with a thin spread of almond butter.
- Herbal tea or water.

### Lunch:

- Whole wheat tortilla wrapped with turkey and avocado.
- Carrot and cucumber sticks with hummus.

### Dinner:

- Steamed broccoli and roasted sweet potatoes with grilled chicken breast.
- Mixed green salad with lemon-tahini dressing.

### Snack:

- Greek yogurt with sliced strawberries.

**Day 2:**

**Breakfast:**

- Smoothie made with banana, unsweetened almond milk, spinach, and a scoop of protein powder.
- Herbal tea or water.

**Lunch:**

- Whole grain bread on the side with lentil soup.
- Mixed green salad with balsamic vinaigrette.

**Dinner:**

- Roasted Brussels sprouts and quinoa pilaf with baked salmon
- Sliced cucumber and tomato salad with olive oil and lemon juice.

**Snack:**

- Apple slices with almond butter.

**Day 3:**

**Breakfast:**

- Almond milk, chia seeds, rolled oats, and sliced strawberries combine to make overnight oats.
- Herbal tea or water.

**Lunch:**

- Quinoa and black bean salad topped with diced avocado and lime dressing
- Handful of mixed nuts.

**Dinner:**

- Brown rice, snap peas, and bell peppers with stir-fried tofu.
- Mixed green salad with lemon-tahini dressing.

**Snack:**

- Cottage cheese with pineapple chunks.

**Day 4:**

**Breakfast:**

- Poached eggs and mashed avocado with whole grain bread.
- Herbal tea or water.

**Lunch:**

- Chicken and vegetable stir-fry with brown rice.
- Sliced bell peppers with hummus.

**Dinner:**

- Baked cod with quinoa and steamed asparagus.
- Mixed green salad with balsamic vinaigrette.

**Snack:**

- Banana slices with almond butter on a rice cake.

**Day 5:**

**Breakfast:**

- Greek yogurt parfait topped with mixed berries and granola.
- Herbal tea or water.

**Lunch:**

- Whole wheat tortilla  with turkey and cheese roll-ups.
- Carrot sticks with hummus.

**Dinner:**

- Vegetable and lentil curry with brown rice.
- Mixed green salad with lemon-tahini dressing.

**Snack:**

- Apple slices with a sprinkle of cinnamon.

**Day 6:**

**Breakfast:**

- Scrambled eggs with diced tomatoes and spinach.
- Whole grain toast topped with a thin spread of almond butter.
- Herbal tea or water.

**Lunch:**

- Tuna salad lettuce wraps with cucumber slices.
- Handful of mixed nuts.

**Dinner:**

- Steamed broccoli and quinoa pilaf with grilled shrimp skewers.
- Mixed green salad with balsamic vinaigrette.

**Snack:**

- Greek yogurt with honey and chopped nuts.

**Day 7:**

**Breakfast:**

- Oatmeal with sliced banana and honey drizzled on top.
- Herbal tea or water.

**Lunch:**

- Chickpea salad with mixed greens, diced bell peppers, cherry tomatoes, and lemon-tahini dressing.
- Sliced cucumber with hummus.

**Dinner:**

- Roasted sweet potatoes and green beans with baked chicken thighs.
- Mixed green salad with balsamic vinaigrette.

**Snack:**

- Cottage cheese with sliced peaches.

# Week Four

**Day 1:**

**Breakfast:**

- Scrambled eggs with spinach and mushrooms.
- Whole grain toast with a thin spread of avocado.
- Herbal tea or water.

**Lunch:**

- Quinoa salad with cherry tomatoes, cucumber, bell peppers, and lemon-tahini dressing.
- Sliced apple with almond butter.

**Dinner:**

- Baked chicken breast with roasted sweet potatoes and steamed green beans.
- Mixed green salad with balsamic vinaigrette.

**Snack:**

- Greek yogurt with honey and sliced strawberries.

**Day 2:**

**Breakfast:**

- Spinach, banana, almond milk, and a scoop of protein powder smoothie.
- Herbal tea or water.

**Lunch:**

- Whole wheat tortilla with turkey and avocado wrap.
- Carrot and celery sticks with hummus.

**Dinner:**

- Roasted Brussels sprouts and quinoa pilaf with baked salmon
- Mixed green salad with lemon-tahini dressing.

**Snack:**

- Cottage cheese with pineapple chunks.

**Day 3:**

**Breakfast:**

- Almond milk, chia seeds, rolled oats, and sliced strawberries combine to make overnight oats.
- Herbal tea or water.

**Lunch:**

- Whole grain bread on the side with lentil soup.
- Mixed green salad with balsamic vinaigrette.

**Dinner:**

- Stir-fried tofu with broccoli, snap peas, and brown rice.
- Sliced cucumber and tomato salad with olive oil and lemon juice.

**Snack:**

- Strawberry slices and almond butter on a rice cake.

**Day 4:**

**Breakfast:**

- Whole grain toast with scrambled eggs and sliced avocado.
- Herbal tea or water.

**Lunch:**

- Chicken and vegetable stir-fry with brown rice.
- Sliced bell peppers with hummus.

**Dinner:**

- Baked cod with quinoa and steamed asparagus.
- Mixed green salad with lemon-tahini dressing.

**Snack:**

- Apple slices with almond butter.

**Day 5:**

**Breakfast:**

- Greek yogurt parfait topped with mixed berries and granola.
- Herbal tea or water.

**Lunch:**

- Whole wheat tortilla with cheese roll-ups and turkey.
- Carrot sticks with hummus.

**Dinner:**

- Vegetable and lentil curry with brown rice.
- Mixed green salad with balsamic vinaigrette.

**Snack:**

- Cottage cheese with sliced peaches.

**Day 6:**

**Breakfast:**

- Scrambled eggs with diced tomatoes and spinach.
- Whole grain toast topped with a thin spread of almond butter.
- Herbal tea or water.

**Lunch:**

- Tuna salad lettuce wraps with cucumber slices.
- Handful of mixed nuts.

**Dinner:**

- Steamed broccoli and quinoa pilaf with grilled shrimp skewers.
- Mixed green salad with lemon-tahini dressing.

**Snack:**

- Greek yogurt with honey and chopped nuts.

**Day 7:**

**Breakfast:**

- Oatmeal with sliced banana and honey drizzled on top.
- Herbal tea or water.

**Lunch:**

- Chickpea salad with mixed greens, diced bell peppers, cherry tomatoes, and lemon-tahini dressing.
- Sliced cucumber with hummus.

**Dinner:**

- Roasted sweet potatoes and green beans with baked chicken thighs.
- Mixed green salad with balsamic vinaigrette.

**Snack:**

- Apple slices with a sprinkle of cinnamon.

# Conclusion

The "Pancreatitis Diet Cookbook for Beginners" provides a thorough and user-friendly guide for anyone coping with the difficulties associated with pancreatitis. This cookbook offers a well selected collection of dishes that not only offer tasty meal options, but also offer insightful information on maintaining and promoting pancreatic health. Even if you are new to cooking, you can confidently produce healthy recipes that are easy on the pancreas with simple, understandable directions.

In addition to dishes, the cookbook provides useful information about how food decisions affect pancreatitis management, including pointers for meal planning, substituting ingredients, and controlling portion sizes. It promotes a proactive attitude to health and well-being by arming you with information and useful tools.

Furthermore, the cookbook offers a wide variety of dishes for breakfast, lunch, dinner, and snacks since it understands how important variety and flavor are to keeping a balanced diet. You can find something to suit every taste and occasion, ranging from hearty soups to filling main meals and decadent desserts.

To sum up, the "Pancreatitis Diet Cookbook for Beginners" is an invaluable resource for anybody seeking improved health. It offers scrumptious dishes together with the information and motivation needed to make wise dietary decisions and promote pancreatic wellbeing.

# Measurement conversion

## Dry Ingredient Conversions

3 teaspoons=1 tablespoon=1/2 ounce=14.3 grams
2 tablespoons=1/8 cup=1 fluid ounce=28.3 grams
4 tablespoons=1/4 cup=2 fluid ounces=56.7 grams
5 1/3 tablespoons=1/3 cup=2.6 fluid ounces=75.6 grams
8 tablespoons=1/2 cup=4 ounces=113.4 grams=1 stick butter
12 tablespoons=3/4 cup=6 ounces=.375 pound=170 grams
32 tablespoons=2 cups=16 ounces=1 pound=453.6 grams
64 tablespoons=4 cups=32 ounces=2 pounds=907 grams

# Liquid Ingredient Conversions

1 cup=8 fluid ounces=1/2 pint=237 ml
2 cups=16 fluid ounces=1 pint=474 ml
4 cups=32 fluid ounces=1 quart=946 ml
2 pints=32 fluid ounces=1 quart=946 ml
4 quarts=128 fluid ounces=1 gallon=3.784 liters
8 quarts=one peck
4 pecks=one bushel
Dash=less than 1/4 teaspoon

# Weight Ingredient conversions

1 ounce = 28 grams
1 pound = 16 ounces
1 pound = approximately 1/2 kilogram
1 kilogram = 1,000 grams
1 kilogram = 2.2 pounds

# The dirty dozen and the clean fifteen

## The Dirty Dozen

These are the twelve fruits and vegetables with the highest levels of pesticide residue, according to EWG's analysis. It's recommended to buy these organic whenever possible to reduce exposure to potentially harmful chemicals. The Dirty Dozen includes:

1. Strawberries
2. Spinach
3. Kale, collard and mustard greens
4. Peaches
5. Pears
6. Nectarines
7. Apples
8. Grapes
9. Bell and hot peppers
10. Cherries
11. Blueberries
12. Green beans

# The Clean 15

These are the fifteen fruits and vegetables with the lowest levels of pesticide residue, making them safer options to buy conventionally grown. While buying organic is always beneficial, these items are less likely to contain significant pesticide residues. The Clean Fifteen includes:

1. Avocados
2. Sweet corn
3. Pineapples
4. Onions
5. Papayas
6. Sweet peas
7. Asparagus
8. Honeydew melons
9. Kiwi
10. Cabbage
11. Mushrooms
12. Mangoes
13. Sweet potatoes
14. Watermelon
15. Carrots